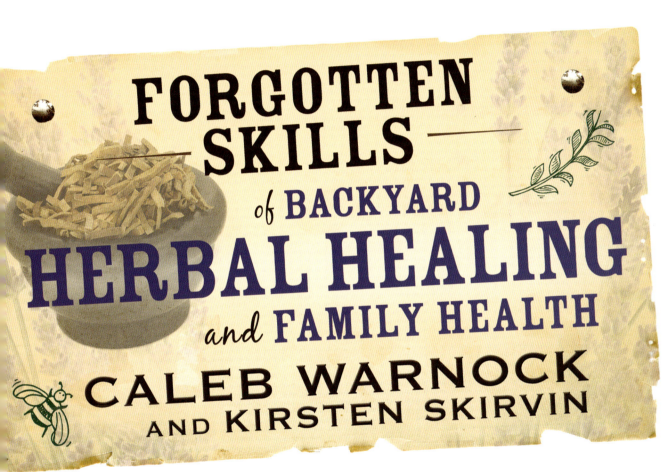

FORGOTTEN SKILLS

of BACKYARD

HERBAL HEALING

and FAMILY HEALTH

CALEB WARNOCK
AND KIRSTEN SKIRVIN

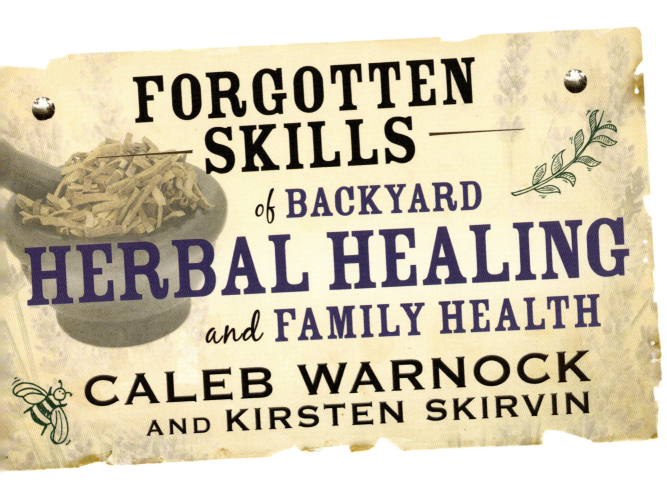

FORGOTTEN SKILLS

of BACKYARD

HERBAL HEALING

and FAMILY HEALTH

CALEB WARNOCK

AND KIRSTEN SKIRVIN

HOBBLE CREEK PRESS

AN IMPRINT OF CEDAR FORT, INC.
SPRINGVILLE, UTAH

ISBN 13: 978-1-4621-1377-4

Published by Hobble Creek Press, an imprint of Cedar Fort, Inc.
2373 W. 700 S., Springville, UT 84663
Distributed by Cedar Fort, Inc., www.cedarfort.com

Library of Congress Cataloging-in-Publication Data

Skirvin, Kirsten, 1963- author.
 Forgotten skills of backyard herbal healing and family health / Kirsten Skirvin and Caleb Warnock.
    pages cm
 Includes bibliographical references and index.
 ISBN 978-1-4621-1377-4
 1. Herbs--Therapeutic use. I. Warnock, Caleb (Caleb J.), 1973- author. II. Title.

 RM666.H33S577 2014
 615.3'21--dc23

                    2014027824

Cover design by Angela Baxter, Rebecca J. Greenwood, and Lacey Hathaway
Page design by Michelle May
Cover design © 2015 by Lyle Mortimer
Edited by Eileen Leavitt

Printed in China

10 9 8 7 6 5 4 3 2 1

DISCLAIMER

Kirsten Skirvin and Caleb Warnock are not medical doctors. The information in this book is not medical advice and should not be treated as such. This book presents time-honored historic herbal and natural methods. You should research and make your own decisions as to your health. The herbal products and methods identified in this book have not been evaluated by the FDA and are not intended to treat or prevent disease. The information provided here is for educational purposes only, and should not be used to diagnose and treat diseases.

In this book you will find a discussion of conditions these products have been used to aid. We are not claiming that the product will cure any of these diseases or that we created them to cure these diseases. We are merely reporting that people have used the product to aid these conditions. Always seek the advice of your physician whenever making healthcare decisions. A licensed medical professional should be consulted for diagnosis and treatment of any and all medical conditions.

CONTENTS

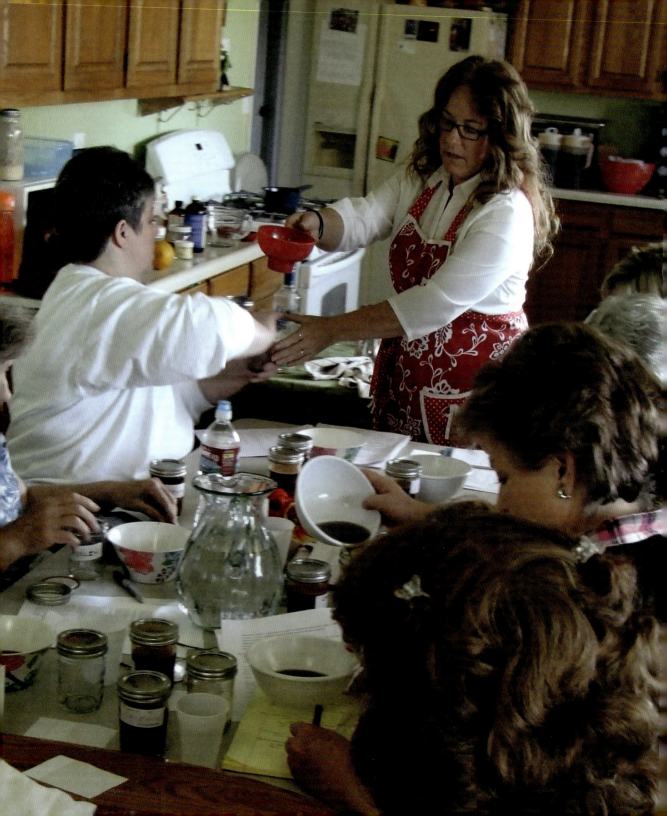

CHAPTER 1

KIRSTEN'S STORY

When I was young, my dad would spend summers with us in the mountains of California. We hiked, backpacked, and picnicked. He enjoyed pointing out the plants and trees around us, giving their names and their native uses. It was so fascinating to know that everything around me had a name and a purpose. These woodland hikes helped me shape how I saw, and continue to see, this amazing planet.

I continued to love the outdoors, and I worked as a wilderness instructor in the southern Utah desert. I learned which herbs were edible and which were poisonous. During that time, I took a wild edibles class in Idaho at the Rabbit Stick Rendezvous. I expected to go on a long hike to find edible and medicinal plants. To my surprise, the teacher stood next to a small pond and pointed out all the wild edibles and medicinal plants for over an hour, without even moving! Can you imagine? I had been fascinated with plants before the class. Afterward, I was convinced this was my calling. I began studying on my own, with small success, and finally became acquainted with the School of Natural Healing in Springville, Utah, where I earned my Master Herbalist certification in 2005.

After I had begun taking classes in herbal medicine, I adopted triplet girls. That brought our children to five, with the girls in between two boys. I wanted to take them to a bonding ropes course. So, we traveled to Utah and participated in a family ropes course activity. One of the activities was to jump off a high pole while saying something amazing. Well, I had always been frightened of that pole but decided that day to do the jump. I was not wholly committed to my cause, and when I jumped, I held on to the rope behind my head to give me the illusion of stability. I grabbed the wrong rope, and it burned through my hand, leaving it shredded. I immediately applied my homemade comfrey salve. I applied it several times a day and kept my hand wrapped to keep it clean. It was interesting to watch as the comfrey left white matter—new cells—all over my hand. Within a week, my hand was completely healed with no scars.

I adopted my youngest at birth. He was nine pounds and five ounces. Though he seemed healthy, he screamed daily from the day he was born. I nursed him with the aid of supplements for a few weeks, but he would vomit after almost every feeding. At one year of age, we took him to a major, reputable medical center, where he was diagnosed with GERD (gastroesophageal reflux disease). They explained that he had to have a fundoplication surgery, which would tie off his esophagus to prevent vomiting, or he could eventually have cancer of the throat. We agreed to the surgery, and they went in and tightened the area between the esophagus and the stomach to prevent regurgitation (GERD). Several days later, he was still trying to throw up. I met with the doctor who informed me that this was now a habit of his, and there was nothing more they could do for him. This was difficult for me to accept. We had just been through major surgery, and my son's poor little body was so tired and sick. We then found a naturopath doctor who, after examining him, stated that he was allergic to milk. She gave us a remedy, we stopped giving him milk, and within twenty-four hours he stopped trying to vomit.

In writing this book, I want you, the reader, to become educated so you can take care of yourself and your family when going to the doctor is not an option. There are many scenarios where this could happen. Use your imagination, and I am sure you could come up with some yourself. We are living in a time when earthquakes, tsunamis, war, and politics have wreaked havoc on our planet. Many have been displaced or have perished in these devastating events. What can we do? We can be prepared. When we are prepared, with herbs stored in case of crises, and the knowledge of how to use them, we are no longer helpless. We become part of the solution.

There are many ways to become acquainted with medicinal herbs, from purchasing them at your local grocer to researching the mysteries of herbs and their uses. In this book, I try to emphasize medicinal herbs you can grow at home or find in your own cupboard or field. Before I moved to Arizona, I lived in a house that had a field across the street. In the field, I could find an abundance of shepherd's purse (to stop hemorrhaging), alfalfa (for nutrition), red clover (for the heart), dock (for the lymph system), dandelion (for liver cleansing and health), gum weed (for coughs and colds), and plantain (to draw out poison). That does not include the trees and plants around my area that were planted with purposes too numerous to include here. I now believe I have a responsibility to learn the local flora in my new home in Arizona and how to grow the herbs I am familiar with. When I look around me, I want to be surrounded by nature's medicine chest.

I believe there is strength and wisdom in planting, harvesting and preparing your own medicinal herbs. Dr. John R. Christopher, founder of the School of Natural Healing, stated he wanted to see an herbalist in every home and a master herbalist in every community. I owe much to this great man and the knowledge and inspiration he passed on to those who had a desire to learn.

My thanks also to the many amazing teachers at the school, the friends who listened to my story, my seven amazing children who helped me memorize my herbs on long walks and who have trusted me with their care, and my wonderfully husband, Steve. I have taught many groups and individuals the wonder of herbs and their uses. I have seen miracles in the lives of those who have applied these principles. There is a moment in our lives when we begin to trust. As you begin to apply the principles that have been taught in this book, you too will come to trust in yourself and in the strength of the smallest herb.

Kirsten Skirvin
April 2014

CHAPTER 2
CALEB'S STORY

For most of my life, I was one of those people who thought herbal medicine was ridiculous at best, and dangerous at worst.

Not anymore.

Earlier this evening, I had the opportunity to practice emergency herbal medicine. I have no one to blame for this "opportunity" but myself.

A year ago, our one-acre backyard pasture had been "mowed" by two cows and a horse. Now, our pasture is empty of animals but full of winter-killed weeds. It is March 10, 2014, and spring weather has arrived. I had been watching the weather reports carefully all day, and I knew a storm would arrive at dusk, so I went out to burn the weeds from our pasture before the storm hit. (It is safest to burn just before a storm so the rain can douse the land.)

Well, the dead weeds were drier than I thought, and the fire was burning well until the storm front hit hard. Our pasture went from peaceful and windless to a 50-mph blast within seconds. The flames jumped ten feet high and headed for my neighbor's backyard barn. I had only a shovel to fight the flames with—no water, and no cell phone to call for help. I was quickly surrounded by flames, breathing smoke, singeing the hair on my head and arms.

I got the fire out, barely. It took every ounce of strength I had.

After putting out all the hot spots, I headed into the house. I've had asthma all my life, but with careful management of my health, I had not needed my inhaler in at least two years—so long that I didn't know where my inhaler was. I had inhaled a huge volume of smoke, and now my lungs were burning. With my lungs tightening rapidly, my ability to breathe was vanishing fast. For all asthma issues, the first line of defense is a hot shower, to clean the body of allergens that are causing inflammation in the lungs. So I took a shower, but my breathing was still getting worse, and I had begun to cough up phlegm. My voice was raspy.

I had to act fast.

I went to my herbal cabinet and got dried oregano stems and leaves and dried peppermint leaves, each harvested from my garden, and elecampane root and lobelia, which I had purchased. I put a teaspoon of each into a cup of water in a pan on the stove, brought it to a boil, turned off the heat, and left the herbs to steep. Normally I would steep my herbs until the tea was cool enough to drink, but in this case, my breathing was so bad there was no time. I held off for three minutes, then sieved the tea, added cold water, and drank down the whole thing.

My relief was immediate. I was able to take my first deep breath since the fire. My lungs relaxed, thanks to the peppermint, which works quickly and wears off quickly, just as the oregano, elecampane and lobelia really begin to work. Fifteen minutes later, my breathing had returned to near normal—comfortable enough for me to do some more work on this *Backyard Herbal Healing and Family Health* book. (As a sidenote, that one dose did the trick for me. I never had to take any more.)

Our six grandkids were all here on that day, and the two four-year-olds had runny noses and coughs. Not wanting that to spread—and also wanting their coughing to loosen—I dosed the five grandkids with a special medicinal tea blend that I created, including horehound, hyssop, echinacea, goldenseal, and marshmallow root. To make it appealing to the kids, I added stevia and lemon juice and told them it was lemonade. They drank it down. Within hours, the coughing was noticeably looser. (I continued this four times a day for the next three days until their coughing and runny noses had stopped.)

I wish I could tell you that I had a wise great-grandmother who taught me a host of herbal wisdom, passing on the hard-won knowledge of previous generations who knew how to gather backyard herbs to help themselves in times of need. But my experience with herbal medicine began late in life, when I discovered that our neighbor, Kirsten Skirvin, was a master herbalist.

Without herbal medicine, I wouldn't be here today—it's probably safe to say that none of us would. We owe all of modern medicine to both the successes and failures of traditional medicine—every single modern and even ground-breaking treatment we have today has its roots in the autodidactic women and men around the world who observed that certain plants had specific healing qualities. They spent their lives learning how to use these herbs through trial and error. If you poke around in your local and family history, it is not hard to find examples of how herbal medicine was used to save lives. Let me share one story particularly important to me.

When my grandmother, Wilhelmina Huntsman Nielson, was six years old in 1930, she came home from school one day to find the house empty and a huge kettle of boiling water on the wood stove. Her mother was preparing to do laundry and had run across the street for a moment. Curious, Wilhelmina climbed up to see what was in the kettle and tipped it over on herself, badly scalding both her legs. In her eighth decade, she still remembered the pain when she told me this story and showed me the scars she had carried all her life.

The closest doctor was fifty miles away in St. George, Utah. There were no cars in those days. But even if a doctor had been handy, there wasn't much a doctor could do that Wilhelmina's grandmother, who lived across the street, couldn't do herself. She put fresh poultices on her granddaughter's legs for weeks, but eventually infection set in. More poultices and prayer were able to draw the infection out, and Grandma lived, though she missed months of first grade. As the infection went away, her older brother, Cannon, carried her to school and back for months until she could walk on her own.

So, you see, without herbal medicine, I wouldn't exist to write this book.

I feel certain the same can be said about every single person on earth—all of us owe a debt of gratitude to those who studied herbs and medicine the hard way and saved lives.

Our family has seen both the best and the worst of modern medicine.

We are not opposed to modern medicine—we are grateful for it. While I wouldn't be here without herbal practitioners, I also wouldn't be alive without modern science. Here is just one example of why: Not many years ago, I absent-mindedly used a pen to scratch just inside my ear, resulting in a tiny tear to the delicate skin, which introduced a rare and deadly bacteria into my body. I was only saved by modern medicine. As I became more and more sick, my wife insisted that I go to the emergency room. The doctor chewed me out for waiting so long, telling me I could have died without potent antibiotics. I could tell you many other such stories. You, the reader, also have similar stories, no doubt.

No, I'm not opposed to modern medicine. But there are two things medicine has been getting very wrong in the past couple decades: it lacks altruism and encourages dependence rather than self-reliance.

Let's start with the lack of altruism. In 1984, when my wife, Charmayne, got pregnant with my fourth stepdaughter, her then-husband had lost his job. They had no insurance and no savings. Because her previous pregnancies and deliveries had been uneventful, Charmayne was considering having the baby at home. When she talked to her doctor about this plan, he felt she would be safer in the hospital. He offered to let her then-husband paint his garage door in exchange for the doctor bill—yes, paint his garage door. The hospital bill was paid anonymously, I suspect by the doctor himself.

This is modern medicine in its highest form. To this day, my wife gets emotional recalling the doctor's generosity.

It could never happen today.

The world has changed for the worse, and it looks doubtful that the pendulum could ever swing back. Today, doctors are more or less owned by healthcare corporations and no longer have the individual authority to place a financially responsible but out-of-work patient in a hospital in exchange for painting a garage—even if this is what is best for the patient. There are two reasons for this:

One, doctors have become the targets of angry people who sue, sometimes with reasonable cause but increasingly without. These lawsuits have forced doctors to carry heavy malpractice insurance premiums. We, the people of the US, have done this. Shame on us.

But there is hope.

Dr. Michael Ciampi of Portland, Maine, announced in 2013 that he would no longer accept insurance as payment, because it freed him "to do what I think is right for the patients," Ciampi told the Bangor Daily News, noting he could now "make house calls and even negotiate discounts for patients with financial hardships." If more doctors were able to do this, that would be real health care reform. That's when we'd see the cost of medicine truly go down."[1]

Second, corporate hospitals and so-called "non-profit" hospitals—where the directors often are paid enormous salaries—now limit the authority doctors have. While my wife's good doctor was able to make a judgment call in 1984, today the same doctor would likely have little or no authority to act outside the bureaucracy of the hospital. Instead, the hospital would have "allowed" my wife to have the baby, and then billed her for many years afterward, at an interest rate equivalent to the worst credit cards. The whole family would have suffered financially, and by the time the bill plus interest was paid, the original charges would likely have doubled or tripled. Meanwhile, the hospital directors take home six-digit salaries. This is not how medicine should be.

Medical care is getting horribly expensive, whether you are the patient or the doctor. Permit me one more example:

My oldest stepdaughter has a rare condition called Addison's disease. Any stressful situation, such as an injury or even the flu, can throw her into an adrenal crisis. Without immediate medical intervention, she will die within hours. In 2004, just out of college, she was working as a contract archaeologist for the state. One day, her paycheck bounced. The contract company apologized, promised payment, and kept the crew working. The next paycheck bounced too. It became apparent the company was bankrupt. My stepdaughter unexpectedly had no job—and then she got sick. She had to be hospitalized twice or she would have died. She said about the first hospitalization, "They told me to put it on my credit card, which I was dumb enough to do. That took forever to pay off. But I didn't have to pay the second hospital bill. The hospital decided to write it off as part of their required charity to maintain non-profit status because I showed I had no money, and I couldn't pay them."

She tried to get insurance, but because she had a preexisting condition, she was repeatedly denied. She was without insurance for about four years, "which is a long, scary, expensive time to be without insurance, and to pay for my medications," she said. "It was over $120 a month for my medications. I was so grateful when Walmart introduced its $4 generics."

It took her many years to pay off the bill from her first hospitalization plus the thousands of dollars of interest. Eventually, she was able to qualify for Medicaid until she found a new job, but she struggled to find a doctor who would accept her as a patient.

"There are few doctors who accept it, and fewer dentists," she said.

The corporations who "own" the doctors will not accept Medicaid patients because the payments are too small compared to the red-tape paperwork storm required to get the money.

We are grateful that her second hospital bill was forgiven by the hospital, and we are even more grateful that today she has a good job working in a medical laboratory, with good health insurance. Nevertheless, her struggles add up to the death of common-sense altruism in the medical community.

Self-reliance was once a hallmark of health care in the home. Today, America is a nation of people waiting for permission from "the people in charge" before any dare make a move to help ourselves to better health.

There is real danger in giving up sovereignty over our health. Giving up is increasingly easy to do. We have developed a relationship with doctors where we are expected to be "dumb"—we go to them with a problem, they tell us to take a pill or have a surgery, and few questions are asked. I have learned the hard way in my life that anytime I feel pressed to give up personal responsibility, I am on the wrong path.

For example, what if the pill maker is paying the doctor—without your knowledge?

"Pharmaceutical companies paid out more than $250 million to some 17,000 doctors and nurses across the country in 2009 and 2010, according to a new database compiled and published by ProPublica, a non-profit investigative journalism group,"[2] reported ABC World News on Oct. 25, 2010.

The ABC News report is just one in a line of investigative reports into this shameful behavior. So far, the real questions about all of this have yet to be answered. If 17,000 doctors are being paid an incentive by a drug company to prescribe pills to you and me—at the rate of a quarter-billion dollars in just two years—we've gone too far. Must we question our doctors? "Excuse me, are you being paid a stipend by the manufacturer of this pill? Whose best interest is being served here? And why in heaven's name would a pill maker need to pay a doctor to prescribe the drugs in the first place?"

"One can't be sure of any corporation if a huge sum of money should be placed before it,"[3] said Eleanor Roosevelt, quoted in *No Ordinary Time*, by Doris Kearns Goodwin.

The same is true of doctors. If you and I genuinely need a pill, or a medical device, or a surgery, there should be no reason in the world that a doctor needs a financial incentive to prescribe it to us. Yet we are only told about these payments to doctors by journalists—the medical community has kept them secret.

Why?

We are left in a situation where we have been taught that we are too "dumb" to participate in our own healthcare decisions—meanwhile, the doctors are secretly accepting what amounts to bribes from pill makers.

We rely on the opinion of doctors and drug makers—after all, they are "the people in charge," and they have our best interests at heart, right? For example, if our doctor prescribes us a pill, we can feel confident that the pill is safe, right? It's been tested, and the government and the doctors—"the people in charge"—say the pill is what is best for us. So we take it.

The irony is that, while modern medicine saves us, it also betrays us—in the form of cost, availability, and ethics. Corporate hospitals and prescription drug makers can help us—if we can afford them, if we can trust them, and many times, only if we can get insurance.

Recently, a family member of mine wrote on Facebook something disparaging about how organic vegetables are a way of duping people into paying extra for food. I should know better than to stir the pot, but I decided to make a comment.

"To people who question buying organic (or growing organic), I say just this: If you're so certain, buy the pesticide and drink it. If you don't want to drink it, why are you feeding it to your kids and putting it in the ground?" I wrote.

To which my family member replied, "The same reason I don't drink bleach, but I clean my things with it."

"Do you spray bleach on your dinner?" I wrote back. "The real issue is this: You get to choose what chemicals you expose your sons to. But your sons don't get to choose the natural consequences that follow."

What herbal medicine does is give regular people back some control of what we ingest as medicine. Like I said before, I was one of those people who thought herbal medicine was ridiculous at best, and dangerous at worst. My experiences with sinus infections helped change my mind.

I have suffered from sinus infections all my life. But around 2008, the infections got out of control—and with the infections came a wave of migraines. I'm not talking about Facebook migraines, where people get on Facebook and post something like, "I sure wish I could get rid of this migraine I've had for two days!" Real migraines are life-threatening. There are a variety of causes, but mine are triggered by internal pressure from inflammation caused by infection. First I would get sick, then I would begin to see halos, and then I would be unable to walk or stand. Any kind of light produced excruciating, unbearable pain. During my last migraine, the pain left me unconscious on the bedroom floor—and when I woke up, I was very disappointed to find out I had not died but would, in fact, continue suffering. Migraines are no joke.

It got to the point when, in 2008, I had a continuous sinus infection. Within a six-month period, I was prescribed four courses of antibiotics, each stronger than the last. The doctor warned me that soon I would be out of antibiotic options because the infection was not being touched by anything but the strongest drugs. I was miserable. I went to see a specialist, who tried to book me for surgery over the phone—before even examining me. Unclear on how the surgery would help me, I called the doctor back to ask some hard questions. Only then did the surgeon admit that the operation would have no real effect on the sinus infections—they would continue, and I would have internal scar tissue, likely making them worse.

Immediately I canceled the surgery.

I was disgusted at the way I had been treated. I felt the surgeon had literally wanted me on the operating room table for his own financial benefit. I was angry. Between my regular doctor and this specialist, it seemed that I had no options. Before being directed to the surgeon, I had seen a new doctor when my regular doctor was not available. The new doctor said a sentence to me that changed my life: "Are you sinus rinsing?"

I had never heard of it. He described to me that you use a squeeze bottle to put salt water up one nostril. The salt water circulates through your sinus and drains out the other nostril. I thought the doctor was a kook. I had dismissed the whole thing at the time, but after literally being out of options, I decided to do some research into sinus rinsing. I was shocked to discover that sinus rinsing had been used to control sinus infections for more than a thousand years. I talked myself into trying it.

Sinus rinsing changed my life. Not only did my sinus infections nearly disappear, but my allergies—which had always plagued me—also became far easier to control. I found that I could avoid colds and influenza most of the time by sinus rinsing religiously whenever there was a sick person in our house—and as anyone with little kids in school knows, they bring home every cold and flu within a thousand miles.

At the same time, I accidentally discovered the health benefits of baking with natural yeast, which cured my esophageal ulcer and helped me lose weight and get back my gut health after so many rounds of antibiotics—a story I tell in my second book, *The Art of Baking with Natural Yeast.*

After all this, there was one evening my wife came home all excited because she had gone to a class sponsored by our local church where our neighbor, Kirsten Skirvin, taught the basic principles of herbal health and healing. The next day, I invited myself over to Kirsten's house, and then she taught two sold-out classes at my kitchen table and taught me all the basics about herbal medicine along the way. Without her, I would not have had the skills to treat my smoke-burned lungs or the grandkids. Kirsten taught my wife and I how to make tinctures, when to harvest herbs, and which herbs she uses for which conditions, and she introduced me to a world of literature about how herbs have been used historically. The first herb book I ever saw belonged to Kirsten.

Today, I know from experience that herbal and traditional medicine has the power to help people like me take back their health. I no longer feel that going to the doctor is my only option. I no longer feel that I'm an unlucky target, just dreading the day the next cough enters the house. I know how to fight bacteria and viruses and how to help people help themselves. I'm nowhere near Kirsten's level of knowledge and ability yet, but I do have the basics for helping myself. I go to the doctor only rarely today. We still have health insurance, but we use it as a last resort.

I wanted to write this book with Kirsten because I'm healthier today than I have ever been in my life. I feel confident in my ability to do many things to help myself at home—often with the herbs straight out of my garden, with little or no cost to me. I have not only been able to help myself and my family, but I can also help many people around me too. Yesterday, my phone rang early in the morning. It was a neighbor calling to say that after decades of suffering, he was ready to try nasal rinsing for the first time. "I want to get rid of the nasal steroids," he said.

Traditional herbal medicine can work hand-in-hand with modern medicine, and there are a growing number of doctors recognizing the need to put safer and more affordable options back into the hands of everyday people like me.

The goal of this book is to introduce the basics of backyard herbal health and healing—how you can help your family, whether in emergencies or in everyday use. We can all get healthier by taking responsibility for our own diet, pills, and medical care. We need to take control by first doing what we can ourselves, discerning and learning what is possible to do for ourselves, before going to doctors—and when we do go to the doctor, we must know our rights and exercise our right to ask questions.

We can do more for ourselves and find peace, and we can do it safely and wisely.

Caleb Warnock
Utah County, Utah
March 18, 2014

Notes

1. Neetzan Zimmerman, "Maine Doctor Slashes Prices by Rejecting Health Insurance," May 29, 2013, accessed October 21, 2014, http://gawker.com/maine-doctor-slashes-prices-by-rejecting-health-insuran-510289623.

2. Kim Carollo, "Pay Dirt: Hundreds of Doctors Earned Big Money from Drug Companies," October 25, 2010, accessed October 21, 2014, http://abcnews.go.com//Health/Wellness/drug-companies-payments-doctors-revealed-database/story?id=11929217.

3. Doris Kearns Goodwin, *No Ordinary Time* (New York: Simon & Schuster, 1994), 60.

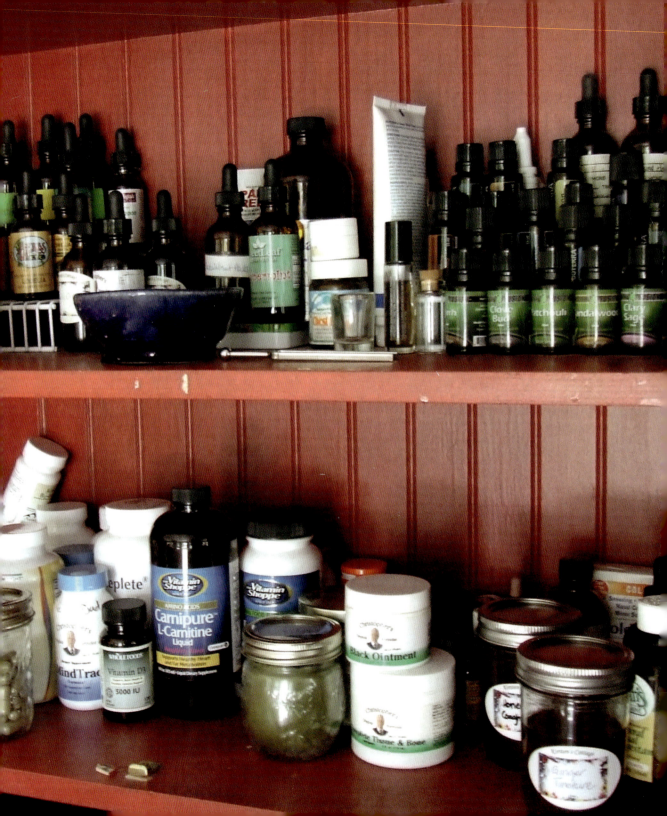

CHAPTER 3
HOW HERBS WORK

There are two bedrock principles at the heart of herbal medicine. The first is that, when it comes to healing and health, we must each decide to save ourselves instead of waiting for someone to save us. The second is that we help the body heal instead of fighting the body.

When Kirsten teaches herbal healing classes, she likes to tell this story:

> ### The Seven Habits of Healthy People
>
> 1. Healthy people change their habits if their habits are making them sick.
>
> 2. Healthy people don't diet. They sustain healthy eating habits.
>
> 3. Healthy people find ways to love moving—skiing, running, or yoga, for example.
>
> 4. Healthy people eschew chemicals and processed foods.
>
> 5. Healthy people cook at home as often as possible using fresh ingredients, avoiding pre-packaged food.
>
> 6. Healthy people make incremental and sustainable changes, never vast changes.
>
> 7. Healthy people make doctors the last line of defense, not the first.

"One time I was sitting in a restaurant and I started choking on spaghetti. I had just kind of sucked it down. My little sister, who was eating with us, said 'That is so gross! Would you stop making that face!' I realized that no one was going to save me. So I dug down into my throat, pulled out the spaghetti, and started breathing again. Sometimes you just have to save yourself."

Unlike prescription medicine, herbal remedies work with your body.

Perhaps the best way to illustrate this is to compare over-the-counter cough syrup and homemade herbal cough syrup. The store-bought stuff is formulated to stop your cough. The problem with this is that coughing is designed to expel toxins from the body. The herbal cough syrup recipe in this book is designed to encourage your body to move mucus out of the body.

"When using herbal remedies, we believe our bodies are coughing for a reason," says Kirsten. "We take a cough syrup that makes our cough productive, i.e., expelling mucus while we cough. We try to assist the body in healing itself."

Caleb and his wife have a friend whose health is failing fast. For the sake of privacy, we'll call this person Sheila. Over the past year, Sheila's life has become filled with doctors, specialists, medical bills, pills and medications, sick leave from work, and opportunities lost because she was forced into bed. Sheila is morbidly obese. Several surgeries and trips to the emergency room have helped in the short term, but the prognosis is not good.

This is painful for us because this person has everything needed for health—all of the answers are at Sheila's fingertips, but Sheila will not lift a finger.

What to do?

Sheila is caught in what I will call a *responsibility trap*.

In the modern world, we are surrounded by responsibility traps. The goal of the people setting the traps is to convince you that you are not responsible because you are a victim. They want you to believe that what is happening to you is outside of your control—that your case is a sad case, a long road. Your job is simply to struggle through.

Meanwhile, the person who set the trap gets rich. You might be tempted to think that I am being cynical, that I am overstating the problem or seeing motives that don't exist. But understanding how responsibility traps work, where to find them, and how to avoid them can give you back your health. And it can help you help the people you love.

So, back to Sheila. Recently, Sheila was taken to the emergency room because she was choking and struggling to swallow and get enough air. Immediately I knew what was wrong. Sheila had an esophageal ulcer. How did I know? Not because I'm psychic. I knew from experience. Fifteen years earlier, I had been rushed from work to the emergency room with the exact symptoms. At first, the doctors thought I was having a heart attack at a very young age. But the real problem was an ulcer in my esophagus, radiating pain through my chest.

So I knew exactly what was happening to Sheila because I used to be Sheila. Fifteen years ago, I was morbidly obese and fighting for my health. I have been where Sheila is.

I can tell you what Sheila's future looks like, because for a long time, it was my future too. Over the next five to ten years, Sheila will continue to see a cascade of doctors. Trips to the emergency room will become annual, and then a couple times a year, and then more. The bills will mount. Hope will not. The number of prescription medications Sheila takes will climb. Symptoms will keep cropping up, demanding more medical intervention. Eventually, Sheila will die prematurely, in her late 50s or early 60s, just like her mother did.

This is Sheila's future. But it doesn't have to be.

More and more Americans are facing a future very much like Sheila's. But there is a way out. We have made doctors our first line of defense. We have reversed their natural role. Doctors should be our last line of defense. Doctors are here to do only what we cannot do for ourselves. When we refuse to do what we can, we force doctors into an untenable position of being responsible for our health. And they can't be. It's not physically possible.

When we take responsbility for our own health, the whole picture changes. This always begins with our diet—the way we eat. What we put in our mouth is a direct sign of our respect—or disrespect—for our health. Whatever we put into our mouth, we will not be able to escape the natural consequences that follow. If we eat right, the natural consequences are good. We are healthy. When we don't, the natural consequences can be brutal, even deadly. Never before in the world have so many people tortured themselves—made themselves sick and ultimately dead—with the food they put into their mouths. When we are young, we feel unlucky if we get sick, and we feel we can eat anything we want. As we get older, we realize there is a direct, immediate connection between what we eat and how we feel.

The 1828 edition of *Webster's American Dictionary of the English Language* gives it to us straight when it defines the word *liberty* like this: "Freedom from restraint, in a general sense, and applicable to the body, or to the will or mind. The body is at liberty when not confined; the will or mind is at liberty when not checked or controlled. A man enjoys liberty when no physical force operates to restrain his actions or volitions."[1]

Eating is one of the best illustrations of the difference between liberty and freedom. When we eat healthy foods, we are not confined by illness. With good health, I am free to be useful to myself, my family, and the community. I am free to hone my talents, polish my intellect, make a positive impact in the world—in short, to be useful to the people around me. Confined by sickness, my freedom gets smaller, until I am dead.

Think of your life as a pie chart of hours. If I am lucky enough to live to age seventy, I could roughly divide up all the hours I've spent in my seventy years like this:

thirty percent = sleeping

ten percent = eating

twenty percent = education

forty percent = freedom to choose

So, back to Sheila. She has forty percent of her lifetime hours to spend freely. This is true for me and you, too. I call this forty percent "time to make myself useful." Every hour we are sick or exhausted of energy is one less hour we can spend to achieve and to be present in our own life. Our achievements might include raising our children, earning a living, making a difference, and helping people.

Time to make ourselves useful is our greatest gift. No one knows how many of these hours he or she will get. We have all mourned when death cuts life short. What if we cut short our own useful hours? We are responsible to protect our health. If we use our liberty carefully, we will be free to spend our healthy hours making ourselves useful. We can do useful work, raise bright and happy children, lend a hand to a neighbor, and influence lives. When we eat ourselves sick, our sickness eats our useful hours.

Ultimately, herbal medicine is about eating ourselves healthy. It starts with good food, but sometimes we need medicine too.

There are two kinds of medicine—preventative and restorative.

Medicinal herbs can be decidedly weak as restorative medicine. After all, if you are bleeding profusely, you are not going to treat that with herbal tea. Modern medicine is invested in being restorative, against the odds. This is not always good for us. My wife has tried without success to convince the kids, who are parents now themselves, that "back in the day"

Preventative Medicine	Restorative Medicine
- builds our immune system	- stops death or significant permanent damage
- boosts our energy and metabolism	- must work against the odds
- circles us with natural protection	- has side effects ("the lesser of two evils")

people did not let their kids do many of the dangerous things we let kids do today, ranging from sports to games to entertainment. Why? Fear of broken bones. Not that many years ago, broken bones often maimed or killed you. Today, few people worry much about broken bones because "we can just go to the doctor." We are confident in the restorative power of modern medicine—so confident that we risk our lives in ways previous generations would have considered reckless. Today, we call it fun.

Medicinal herbs have some restorative power, but they pale in comparison to modern medicine. So who cares about medicinal herbs, right? They are surely of little value in our modern day. They are outmoded, archaic dinosaurs. Tired. Irrelevant. Modern medicine wins, hands down.

Right?

On March 16, 2005, a team of scientists working with the US National Institutes of Health called a press conference to announce something remarkable. "Over the next few decades, life expectancy for the average American could decline by as much as five years unless aggressive efforts are made to slow rising rates of obesity. . . . The US could be facing its first sustained drop in life expectancy in the modern era."[2]

Think about it for a moment. In every generation before us, science has worked to increase our lifespan. Our gift to the upcoming generation? Cutting their lives short. Despite every modern advance, we have failed the only test that matters. We are stealing short the useful hours of our children.

Has restorative medicine failed us? No. We have failed preventative medicine. Combined with good nutrition, medicinal herbs are preventative medicine. Here's how to use them:

STEP 1. STOP ACUTE ILLNESS FROM BECOMING CHRONIC

Whenever you are trying to tamp down and control illness in your own home, it is important to know the difference between acute sickness and chronic sickness. Acute illness is associated with the sudden onset of symptoms, such as the 24-hour flu. Chronic illness is an ongoing illness or condition like diabetes or neuromuscular disease. If an illness is not handled in the acute stage, it can become chronic. For example, a cold can lead to bronchitis, which, in turn, can lead to pneumonia. Or strep throat, left untreated, can become scarlet fever. The goal of any medicine, herbal or otherwise, is to keep acute illness from becoming chronic.

Whenever we speak of illness, and the desire to treat it, think of the following mantra taught to Kirsten by Sandra K. Livingston Ellis in her master herbalist program: "You must be stronger than the illness, or the illness wins."

A drop of an herb that has healing properties, if given sporadically and with the hope that something will occur on its own, will not eradicate illness. To win, you must be more determined to create homeostasis, or internal stability, than the illness is determined to cause a disruption of your health. Winning back your internal stability will take time, patience, and work. Herbs, above all, are food the body needs to heal itself. So, feed the body, and trust in its ability to heal.

Herbs in the proper amounts are food. Your body takes what it needs from them to regenerate.

Be prepared to give herbs time to work in your system. Some things work fast, like lobelia, peppermint, and cayenne. Others need hours, or even several days of doses, to accumulate enough power for your body to break the herb down and let the medicine go to work—for example, onions, garlic, and pine sap.

STEP 2: LEARN YOUR "BIO-INDIVIDUALITY"

Caleb has a nutritionist friend who teaches people that part of the goal of permanently improving your health is to claim and study your "bio-individuality." This term simply means that what works—or doesn't work—for one person is not always the same for everyone else.

Each of us has a unique bio-personality. Caleb is allergic to bananas, raw tomatoes (cooked are fine), cherries, penicillin, and sulfa drugs. He is so allergic to ibuprofen that a single dose lands him in the emergency room. Caleb also has a visceral reaction to garden sweet peppers. Why? Who knows? Some of it is genetic—the tomato allergy runs strongly in his family. Another strong genetic trait that has plagued Caleb is insomnia. His grandfather and many of his cousins suffered from it. Controlling insomnia has taken years to learn. All of these traits are part of Caleb's bio-identity. Each of us is different.

For you, the reader, one medicinal herb might become your favorite because it helps you control some chronic allergy or other condition in your life. You might find that your body has a special relationship with chamomile for calming and helping you sleep—or it might be valerian or skullcap or St. John's Wort. For some people, any of these might work fine. Some people might not like the taste of a particular herb and choose to use another with similar properties. No one can make these decisions for you—only

you will be able to "read" your body's relationship with different herbs.

Learning to read your own body is something most people need to do better. As Caleb's nutritionist friend likes to say, we would all be healthier if we would pay attention to our body's signals and needs and learn to make more decisions about our health based on internal or personal analysis instead of, for example, the "cures" or diets that we see floating around the Internet.

STEP 3: LEARN TO COMPARE AND CONTRAST HERBS

There is an important lesson that must be understood. Many herbs have similar properties. These herbs can be grouped into categories:

- Diuretics, which are herbs that help with the urinary tract.

- Alteratives, which are herbs that alter the blood stream.

- Expectorants or demulcents, which are herbs that clean out the body.

- Nervines, also called antispasmodics, which relieve stress.

- Diaphoretics, which help you sweat.

- Astringents, which tighten the body (pores, gums, muscles, and skin, for example).

- Emmenagogues, which help with reproduction.

- Stimulants, which enhance or produce action in the body.

- Cathartics, which help with defecation, or discharge of feces.

There are many different herbs within each of these types, and some herbs belong to two or more of these categories.

Kirsten has familiarized herself with about one hundred herbs. "Are there other herbs on the planet that are comparable to the ones I know? Yes, there are. I am always fascinated to learn more and to constantly study the findings of herbalists throughout the world. I may try a new herb, or I may not. Knowing how the body works and what herbs will help it work better is the ultimate goal for any who are concerned about their own health and the herbs that can be grown in their own backyard. "

STEP 4. TEACH OTHERS

All the medicinal knowledge in the world won't do any good if you are the "practitioner" in your home and you become acutely ill.

At one point, Kirsten had whooping cough and was so sick that she couldn't take care of herself. "I would suggest making a list of illnesses and the herbs you prefer to cure them. Make sure you let your family know where that list is." This book will help you build the foundations of such a list.

Teaching the basics to those around us is important so they can save us when we need them to. But this also helps them on the journey toward becoming self-reliant adults who are confident in their ability to take care of themselves and their families in times of sickness instead of relying on others to make decisions for them at every step.

STEP 5. BE PREPARED

Recently, Caleb got a phone call late at night from a family member who was sick. The caller lived two hours away from Caleb and had no herbs in his home. The herb-selling stores nearest to the caller had long-since closed. This lack of preparedness is something ingrained in us by the pharmaceutical industry—we have become accustomed to a pattern of developing a sickness, then visiting a doctor or emergency room, and then going to a pharmacy. Late night or weekend? No problem—there are 24-hour pharmacies across the country. This pattern does not allow us to prepare before sickness sets in. Ideally, herbal medicine should be different.

We would encourage you to keep a small supply on hand of each of the herbs mentioned in this book. Tinctures take at least two weeks to mature and should be at the ready—tinctures are not something you wait to begin preparing once you get sick.

The same is true of growing herbs, making herbal teas, and practicing herbal remedies. Caleb has written several popular books on self-reliance, and he continues to be amazed at the number of people who want to put seeds into their freezer "in case they need them one day." The day of crisis is not the day to start the process of becoming self-reliant—that is too late. The same is true of practicing herbal medicine. Now is the time to practice. The goal is to practice when you have options so that you are confident and prepared in the day of need.

Notes

1. *Webster's Dictionary 1828—Online Edition*, s.v. "liberty," accessed October 21, 2014, http://webstersdictionary1828.com/.

2. "Obesity Threatens to Cut U.S. Life Expectancy, New Analysis Suggests," NIH News, March 16, 2005, accessed October 21, 2014, http://www.nih.gov/news/pr/mar2005/nia-16.htm.

CHAPTER 4
WHERE TO GET MEDICINAL-GRADE HERBS

I deally you should grow your own medicinal herbs. If you cannot grow your own, you can purchase dried medicinal herbs from SeedRenaissance.com or at your local herb store.

The self-reliant method of growing your own backyard herbs has many advantages

1. *You know where your herbs have been.* You know they are organic and have not been treated with pesticides or herbicides because you are the one who grew them. You know exactly how fresh they are, because you are the one who harvested them.

2. *While most dried medicinal herbs are not expensive, growing your own is virtually free.* Many medicinal herbs are perennial (hyssop, catnip, peppermint, and horehound, just to name a few), meaning they come back year after year. And many of those that are annual or biennial, such as chamomile and mullein, reliably self-seed. For the most part, once you have medicinal herbs growing on your property, you will have a supply for many years to come.

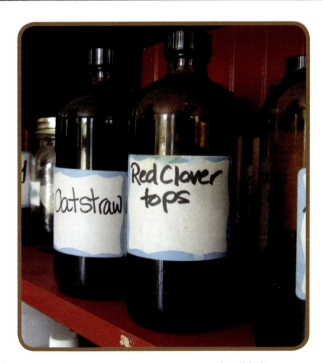

3. *Growing your own means you are less likely to run out of critical herbs.* In fact, you may have enough to share. Hyssop is one of Caleb's favorite medicinal herbs, and it likes to slowly spread as it grows, so you can take starts and give them to friends and

family. As you get more practice at using medicinal herbs, you will know how much you need to harvest and dry for your own use so that you never run out, and you never have to run to the store.

4. *Most herbs are easy to grow.* This is another reason they have been used for thousands of years. Caleb lives at an altitude of five thousand feet in the Rocky Mountains and he has many herbs in his backyard garden, including mullein, lemon balm, chamomile, hyssop, horehound, echinacea, oregano, calendula, red raspberry (leaves are used medicinally), pine trees, and alfalfa. Some medicinal herbs grow wild in Caleb's yard, including mallow, plantain, comfrey, dock, and red clover.

5. *Self-grown herbs have not been irradiated.* Many fresh and dried foods sold in stores today have been subjected to a process called irradiation, which uses low levels of nuclear radiation to sterilize fruits, vegetables and herbs.[1] This sterilization is used to protect people from some of the bacteria and viruses that are increasingly common as a result of eating mass-produced food. Irradiation can destroy at least some part of the medicinal properties of herbs, and it is known to destroy a percentage of the nutrients in fruits and vegetables.

WHERE TO GET SEEDS FOR MEDICINAL HERBS?

When choosing seeds for medicinal herbs, an abundance of caution is required. There are now many pseudo-herbs that have been hybridized to make them more showy for flower bed plantings, but in the process, the herbs have lost much of their medicinal power. The best medicinal herbs are those that grow in their natural form: non-hybridized and never genetically modified.

It is terribly important that medicinal herbs remain in the public domain instead of being owned or patented by corporations. Hybrids are corporately owned and patented, which means it is not legal to sell seeds or starts of those plants, and some companies, such as Monsanto, have been aggressive in taking everyday people to court for even saving the seeds of some trademarked and patented plants. For thousands of years, anyone who wanted to grow medicinal herbs or harvest the seeds or sell or share the seeds has had that legal right. Today, that legal right is threatened by hybrids and genetically modified seed, even as those qualities erode the medicinal quality of the plants. When purchasing medicinal herb seeds, be sure the seller guarantees the seeds as being medicinal in quality.

Some of the best examples of pseudo-herbs are echinaceas and calendulas. The natural medicinal qualities of echinacea have been nearly destroyed in the quest to create new hybrid and genetically modified color variations of this beautiful flower. The medicinal part of the echinacea plant is the root. Natural echinacea, also called purple coneflower, has a purple flower the size of your hand. Hybrids now come in a rainbow of colors—white, green, yellow, orange, red, and many pastels. They are stunning and beautiful, but the plants are extremely weak. True echinacea is a hardy plant that withstands sub-zero temperatures to grow back year after year. Most hybrids are so weak that they do not withstand harsh winters, in Caleb's experience. Hybrids are self-suiciding plants, designed by the manufacturer NOT to produce true seeds. On top of this, growers charge top dollar for hybrid plands and seeds. A single hybrid echinacea at a nursery can cost twenty-five dollars.

If growing your own herbs is not an option for you, ask around for friends who might be growing them. Most of the time, herbalists are happy to share the harvest, especially if you are willing to do some of the harvesting yourself. Many herbalists grow more than they need in a single year. Caleb regularly gives away starts of oregano, lemon balm and other plants in the spring to friends and neighbors who want them.

Caleb's seed company, SeedRenaissance.com, has a large selection of guaranteed medicinal herb seed, many of which are difficult to find.

At SeedRenaissance.com, every seed is guaranteed pure and true, never hybrid, never GMO, never patented, and never corporate-owned. Using a worldwide network of gardeners, Caleb literally searches the globe for the last seeds of important historic varieties, like perennial wheat, and vanishing medicinal herbs. He is single-handedly keeping alive many critical heirloom varieties. You can read about this in his other *Forgotten Skills* books. For every common heirloom sold at SeedRenaissance.com, he has grown and tested 30–40 other varieties. He evaluates how these varieties perform in an organic garden, without petro-chemical fertilizer, pesticides, or herbicides. He evaluates earliness, flavor, production, storage, cold-soil tolerance, winter harvest ability, self-seeding capacity, and more. At SeedRenaissance.com you can find seeds for the following, and more:

- Anise
- Astragalus
- Black Cohosh
- Calendula (high-resin true medicinal)
- Comfrey
- Costmary
- Elecampane
- Feverfew

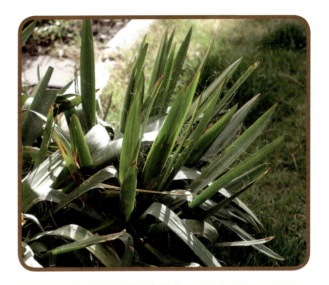

A healthy yucca plant used for making soap

- German Chamomile
- Horehound
- Hyssop
- Lavender
- Lemongrass
- Licorice
- Lobelia
- Ma Huang
- Medicinal-grade Cayenne Peppers
- Mormon Tea
- Mullein
- Oregano
- Peppermint
- Plantain
- Propolis (medicinal product of beehives)
- Self-Heal

- Soapwort (used for making homemade soap)
- Spearmint
- St. John's Wort
- Stevia
- Valerian
- Yarrow
- Yucca (used for making homemade soap)

Each of these varieties is guaranteed to be medicinal quality, sustainably harvested, open-pollinated, pure and true, and not genetically modified or hybrid. At SeedRenaissance.com you will also find full information about how to grow the seeds, how to harvest them, which parts of the plants are used medicinally, and examples of how Caleb uses them. SeedRenaissance.com also features a full line of culinary herb seeds, vegetable seeds, and dried medicinal herbs for home use, both cut and sifted natural herbs and natural herbs that have been ground into powder.

Plants like white yarrow and wild carrot (Queen Anne's lace) look similar but are used for different purposes. Be careful what you harvest!

WILDCRAFTING MEDICINAL HERBS FOR HOME USE

Wildcrafting is the art of going into nature to find medicinal herbs for harvesting. While wildcrafting is a time-honored tradition, there are some concerns:

1. *Sustainability*. As herbal remedies become more and more popular, the human pressure on wild plant stocks increases. Goldenseal is one of the most important of all medicinal herbs because the powder made from the roots of this plant has powerful antibiotic and antiviral qualities. Goldenseal is being used more and more at home and in commercial herbal preparations. Unfortunately, goldenseal has also become one of the prime examples of wild plants being overharvested in nature. When too many people want the same wild herb, the very existence of these important plants is threatened, and herbalists are now speaking out, trying to keep these plants from disappearing from the wild. The answer to all of this is simple—grow and harvest in your own backyard. When we grown our own, we reduce the pressure on Mother Nature.

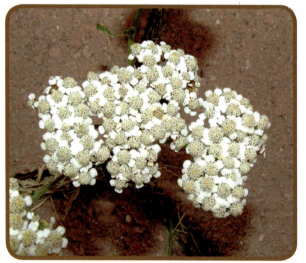

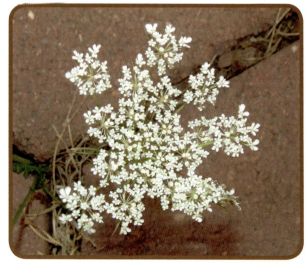

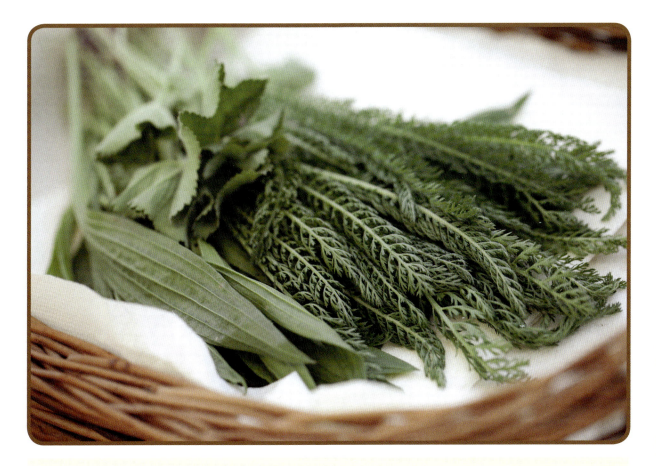

Plantain, yarrow, and lady's mantle. Herbs like this are best picked fresh and then dried for medicinal use.

2. *Safety*. Almost every plant in nature has a look-alike, and this is certainly true of medicinal herbs. Anytime someone without experience attempts to harvest wild herbs, they are taking the risk that they could mistake one of nature's look-alikes for the real thing. Hemlock and Queen Anne's lace are a great example. Hemlock is highly poisonous, and it looks very much like Queen Anne's lace—and even real Queen Anne's lace can be dangerous when used incorrectly. So you can see that "casual" collecting in the wild can be deadly without appropriate training.

Kirsten has an interesting story about working at This Is The Place Heritage Park in Utah.

"I was approached by a young man who was very concerned about the hemlock growing near the schoolhouse," she says. "He suggested we go over and rip out all the hemlock because even the smell could cause harm to children. He had been sent to me because his concern had caused an alarm. I did not quite understand why he was upset, because I was very familiar with the area and had not seen any hemlock or any other dangerous plant. He said that he had been taking a biology class and was convinced he was right. Well, I am glad he was concerned. We must be ever watchful of the volunteer plants that grow around us. However, in this case there was no

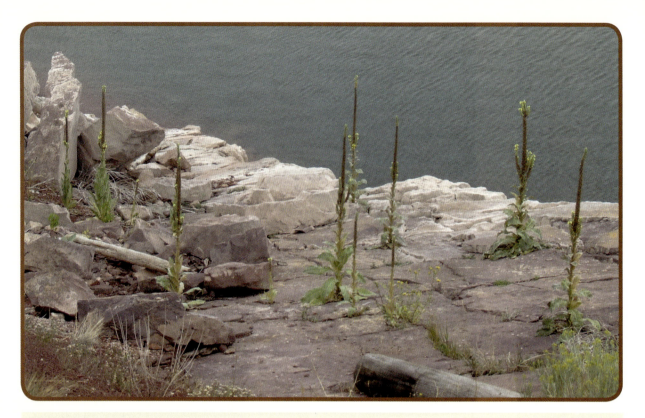

Wild mullein is commonly found in the Rocky Mountains. The leaves of the second year are used medicinally.

hemlock on the site. He had mistaken the Queen Anne's lace for the hemlock. Queen Anne's lace is a beautiful perennial flower with a small black dot in the very center of each."

At the very least, anyone who is going into nature to harvest medicine should go with an experienced herbalist with years of experience in identifying and harvesting from the wild. It is never enough to simply look at some pictures on the Internet, or in a book, and then set out into the woods, desert, or ditch bank to find your own medicine. Never harvest a wild plant unless you know for certain what you are taking, and you have the assistance of an expert.

The answer to this concern, again, is simple. Growing your own medicinal herbs from guaranteed seeds removes any guesswork so that you know exactly what plants you have.

3. *Preserving genetic stocks.* Wild medicinal plants are an important "genetic bank" for herbs. Most of the vegetables we eat today have been improved over centuries to make them bigger, better-tasting, and even more nutritious—carrots are a prime example, and you can read about the history of carrots in Caleb's first *Forgotten Skills* book. But this husbandry is not true for most medicinal herbs. Instead of being improved by humankind, medicinal herbs today are often pretty much exactly the same plants that have been growing wild since the beginning of time. You would never find a big, crisp, orange carrot growing in the wild, but you will find mullein, mallow, yarrow,

plantain, and many other herbs growing wild and filled with medicinal power all on their own. Medicinal plants have developed their power and attributes in nature, and while it is valuable to grow them in our backyard gardens, the genetic stocks of these important plants should remain wild and vigorous so that our backyard plants and medicinal herb seed crops can be boosted by occasionally mixing in wild genetic stock for vigor.

If you do decide to wildcraft your herbs, here are some rules to follow

1. *Be responsible.* Never take more than one-quarter of the plants in a single area. Wild plants must self-perpetuate to survive, so it is critical that we don't take so much that the long-term survival of the patch you have found is in doubt after you harvest.

2. *Take an expert with you.* Never guess at what you are harvesting. Never use a photograph as your guide.

3. *Make sure you have permission to harvest.* It is not legal to harvest anything from private land without permission. It is also illegal to harvest herbs from many public lands. Before harvesting, be sure you know that you have permission not only to be on the land, but also to remove herbs or seeds.

4. *Make sure the herbs are clean.* Caleb has a neighbor and friend who is famous for collecting wild food on walks and bike rides in Caleb's neighborhood. But she is careful to make sure that she picks only in areas where she knows the plants are free from pesticides and herbicides, whether from homeowners or local farmers. Any plant you harvest should be free of toxins and at the peak of health.

5. *Avoid roadsides.* Cars produce carcinogenic residues from their exhaust and the wearing away of rubber tires. These residues end up on roadside plants and are likely far more toxic than herbicides and pesticides.

Notes

1. J. H. Diehl, "Combined Effects of Irradiation, Storage, and Cooking on the Vitamin E and B1 Levels of Foods," *Food Irradiation* 10 (April 14, 1967): 2–7.

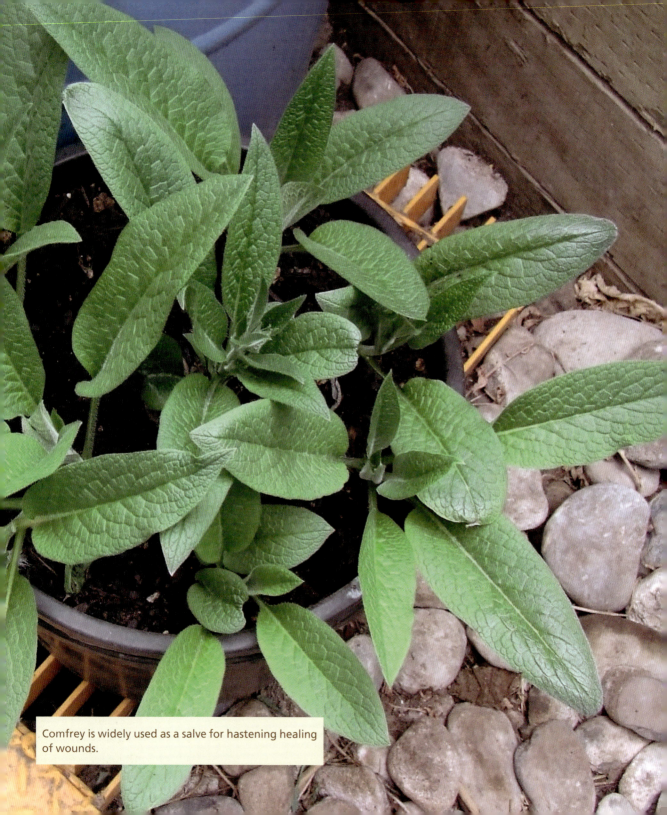

Comfrey is widely used as a salve for hastening healing of wounds.

CHAPTER 5
HOW TO HARVEST, DRY, AND STORE HERBS

When harvesting herbs, the goal is always to pick them at the peak of their potency. The best time to harvest is specific to each individual herb. Harvesting herbs when they are weak will not produce good medicine. For some plants, this means waiting until they flower. For others, it means harvesting before they flower. For yet others, it means digging up the roots either as the plant sprouts in spring, or after the plant dies back in the fall.

Here is a list of the peak times to harvest some common medicinal herbs and the parts of the plant that should be harvested, courtesy of SeedRenaissance.com. These are more common herbs that are used by beginners and experts. This list is not exhaustive, but is intended as a resource for those who are beginning to become familiar with medicinal herbs.

Anise
Pimpinella anisum

This sweet, licorice-flavored herb has been used for centuries for tea, candy making, and for flavoring the famous Italian pizzelle cookies. This is anise official, not star anise. The seeds are the part of the plant used both medicinally and in culinary preparations. Plant directly in the garden soil in fall or early spring, as soon as the soil can be worked. Anise does not like to be grown in pots. It grows annually. Anise is taken internally for upset stomach, flatulence, runny nose, and as an expectorant, diuretic, and appetite stimulant. Anise is also used to increase lactation, induce menstruation, dysmenorrhea, facilitate birth, increase libido, and treat symptoms of 'male menopause.' It can also be used for seizures, nicotine dependence, insomnia, asthma, and constipation. Externally, anise is used for lice, scabies, and psoriasis treatment.[1]

Astragalus
Astragalus membranaceus, recently changed to *Astragalus propinquus*

This medicinal flower is perennial to zone six. The root of four-year-old plants is harvested in the autumn, dried, and then boiled in tea. It is used to improve the immune system and to fight respiratory ailments and heart disease. In Chinese medicine, it is reportedly called Yellow Leader (Huang Qi) because the root is yellow and the plant is highly valued as medicine. This plant likes full sun and well-drained soil with lots of sand and stone. Rub seeds with sandpaper and plant directly in garden in the spring. Barely cover seed and keep seeds moist until germination, which will take one to three weeks. Astragalus is taken internally for common cold, upper respiratory infections, nasal allergies, and swine flu; to strengthen and regulate the immune system; for fibromyalgia, anemia, HIV/AIDS, chronic fatigue syndrome (CFS), chronic nephritis, and diabetes; as an antibacterial, antiviral, tonic, liver protectant, anti-inflammatory, and antioxidant; as a diuretic, a vasodilator, and a hypotensive agent. Externally, astragalus is used as a vasodilator and to speed healing. In combination with *Ligustrum lucidum* (glossy privet), astragalus is used orally for treating breast cancer, cervical cancer, and lung cancer.[2]

Black Cohosh
Cimicifuga racemosa; Actaea racemosa

This herb is a perennial. The root is the part used medicinally. It prefers moist loamy soil and grows only in shade. Sow seeds in the fall for spring germination. Black cohosh is taken internally to induce labor in pregnancy and treat symptoms of menopause, premenstrual syndrome (PMS), dysmenorrhea, nervous tension, dyspepsia, rheumatism, fever, sore throat, and cough. It is also used as an insect repellent and as a mild sedative. Externally, black cohosh is used for acne, mole and wart removal, improving appearance of the skin, and rattlesnake bites.[3]

Calendula (high resin true medicinal)
Calendula officinalis

This herb is an annual. It requires forty to fifty days to achieve maturity. It also prefers full sun. Barely cover the seed, and keep it moist and warm until germination, which takes about a week. Flower petals are used medicinally. Stems and leaves may also be used. Pick flowers after the dew dries and use fresh or dry for later. Calendula flower is taken internally as an antispasmodic, to initiate menstrual periods, to reduce fever, for treating cancer, and for inflammation of oral and pharyngeal mucosa. Calendula has also been used orally for gastric and duodenal ulcers and dysmenorrhea. Externally, calendula flower is used as an anti-inflammatory and for poorly healing wounds and leg ulcers. It is also used topically for nosebleeds, varicose veins, hemorrhoids, proctitis, and conjunctivitis.[4]

Medicinal-grade Cayenne Peppers (capsicum)
Capsicum frutescens

This garden pepper is widely used to bring heat to the body for treating colds, flu, and pain. Start the seeds indoors six to seven weeks before your last frost date. Barely cover seed with soil, press soil firmly, and keep moist until the seed sprouts, which usually takes about two weeks. The red fruits, ripe and dried,

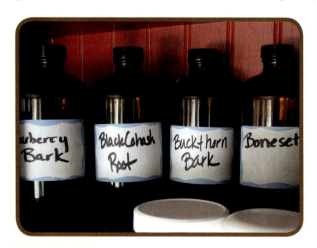

are the parts used medicinally, usually ground into a powder. Transplant outdoors only in hot weather. Cayenne is taken internally for upset stomach, flatulence, colic, diarrhea, cramps, toothache, poor circulation, excessive blood clotting, seasickness, swallowing dysfunction, alcoholism, malaria, fever, hyperlipidemia, and prevention of heart disease. Externally, cayenne is taken for shingles pain relief, osteoarthritis, rheumatoid arthritis, post-herpetic neuralgia, trigeminal neuralgia, diabetic neuropathy, back pain; post-surgical neuralgia, prurigo nodularis, HIV-associated neuropathy, and fibromyalgia; for muscle spasms relief, as a gargle for laryngitis, and as a deterrent to thumb-sucking or nail biting. Cayenne is taken in the nose for nasal allergies, seasonal allergies, migraine headache, cluster headache, sinonasal polyposis, and sinusitis.[5]

Comfrey
Symphytum officinale

Comfrey is widely used as a salve for hastening healing of wounds. Comfrey is perennial, and it spreads and can monopolize an area. Grow comfrey in a pot buried in your garden to keep it from spreading everywhere. It prefers full sun to part sun in sandy or clay soil. Plant the seed just under the surface and press the soil. Germination takes two to four weeks, and the soil must be warm during this time. Comfrey is a prolific producer of large leaves, making it a favorite for people who make their own garden compost. Internally, comfrey is used as a tea for gastritis, ulcers, excessive menstrual flow, diarrhea, bloody urine, persistent cough, pleuritis, bronchitis, cancer, angina, as a gargle for gum disease, and pharyngitis.

Comfrey is used externally for ulcers, wounds, joint inflammation, bruises, rheumatoid arthritis, phlebitis, gout, and bone fractures.[6]

Elecampane
Inula helenium

This is a self-seeding perennial. It likes rich soil that is wet and likes sun to part-shade. This is a large plant. The roots are the part used medicinally. Sow in spring. Barely cover the seed. Keep warm and in the light until germination, which takes about two weeks. Elecampane is taken internally as an expectorant, antitussive, and diaphoretic; for diseases of the respiratory tract; as an anthelmintic; for improving stomach function; as a diuretic; and for asthma, bronchitis, whooping cough, cough associated with tuberculosis, nausea, and diarrhea.

In foods and beverages, elecampane is used as a flavoring ingredient. In other manufacturing processes, elecampane is used as a fragrance component in cosmetics and soaps.[7]

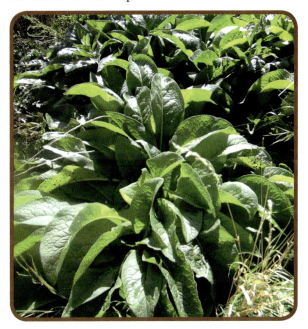

Often used as a salve, Comfrey leaves also make great composting materials.

Feverfew
Tanacetum parthenium

Feverfew is used to treat fevers, migraine headaches, and mild rheumatoid arthritis. This herb prefers well-drained soil. The stems, leaves, and flowers are used medicinally. Sow seed in spring by pressing firmly to soil. Keep moist until seed sprouts in one to two weeks. Internally, feverfew is taken for fever, headaches, prevention of migraines, menstrual irregularities, arthritis, psoriasis, allergies, asthma, tinnitus, vertigo, nausea, vomiting, infertility, anemia, cancer, common cold, earache, liver disease, prevention of miscarriage, muscular tension, orthopedic disorders, swollen feet, diarrhea, and dyspepsia, including indigestion and flatulence. Externally, feverfew is used to treat parasites and toothache and as an antiseptic, insecticide, general stimulant and tonic.[8]

German Chamomile
Matricaria recutita

This is used to make chamomile tea, which has a calming, soothing effect. Chamomile is a reliable self-seeding annual flower. The flowers are the parts used medicinally. These take eighty days to achieve maturity. Sow in spring or autumn and press into the soil firmly. Sprouts in one week. Harvest flowers in early flowering stage and dry to use for making soothing tea. An excellent self-seeder! Internally, German chamomile is taken for flatulence, travel sickness, nasal membrane inflammation, nasal allergies, nervous diarrhea, attention-deficit/hyperactivity disorder (ADHD), fibromyalgia, restlessness, insomnia, gastrointestinal (GI) spasms, colic, inflammation of the GI tract, GI ulcers associated with nonsteroidal anti-inflammatory drugs (NSAIDs) and alcohol consumption, and as an antispasmodic for menstrual cramps. Externally, German chamomile is used for hemorrhoids; mastitis; leg ulcers; pressure ulcers; peristomal skin lesions; skin, anogenital, and mucous membrane inflammation; atopic dermatitis; and bacterial skin diseases, including those of the mouth and gums. It is also used topically for treating or preventing chemotherapy- or radiation-induced oral mucositis. As an inhalant, German chamomile is used to treat inflammation and irritation of the respiratory tract. In foods and beverages, German chamomile is used as flavor components. In manufacturing, German chamomile is used in cosmetics, soaps, and mouthwashes.[9]

Horehound (white)
Marrubium vulgare

This is a perennial. The stems and leaves are the parts used medicinally. It prefers full sun and fast-draining soil with dry conditions. Scrape the seed with sandpaper, press onto a soil surface, and keep moist until germination, which takes up to three weeks. Keep seedlings warm. White horehound is taken internally for loss of appetite, cough, bronchitis, respiratory tract membrane inflammation, whooping cough, asthma, tuberculosis, indigestion, bloating and flatulence, diarrhea, jaundice, debility, liver and gallbladder complaints, and painful menstruation, and as a laxative, anthelmintic, diuretic, and sweat inducer. Externally, white horehound is used for skin damage, ulcers, and wounds. In manufacturing, white horehound extract is used as flavoring in foods and beverages, and as an expectorant in cough syrups and lozenges.[10]

Hyssop
Hyssopus officinalis

This herb is a perennial. Leaves, stems and flowers are the parts used medicinally. It likes moist, rich

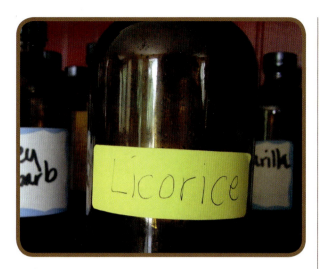

soil in sun or shade. Press into soil and keep moist until germination, which takes about a week. Water only gently, so as not to dislodge germinating roots. Will slowly spread to form a patch if given regular water, so keep in pots or inside a border for control. Hyssop is taken internally for liver and gallbladder conditions, intestinal inflammation, coughs, the common cold, respiratory infections, sore throat, asthma, urinary tract infection, flatulence, colic, anorexia, poor circulation, HIV/AIDS, dysmenorrhea, and for digestive and intestinal problems. Externally, hyssop is used as a gargle; in baths to induce sweating; and for treating skin irritations, burns, bruises, and frostbite. In foods, hyssop oil and extract are used as a flavoring. In manufacturing, hyssop oil is used as a fragrance in soaps and cosmetics.[11]

Licorice Official
Glycyrrhiza glabra

This is a perennial herb. It prefers alkaline soil. Rub seed with sandpaper before planting in spring. Germination takes one to two weeks. The roots are the parts used in medicine to treat respiratory illness, and in culinary preparations for their strong licorice flavoring. Caleb likes to add licorice to most herbal medicinal teas because it gives a naturally sweet, delicious flavor. Roots can be harvested beginning in autumn of the second year and thereafter. Licorice is taken internally for gastric and duodenal ulcers, sore throat, bronchitis, chronic gastritis, dyspepsia, colic, menopausal symptoms, primary adrenocortical insufficiency, cough, osteoarthritis, osteoporosis, systemic lupus erythematosus (SLE), and for bacterial and viral infections. It is also used orally for cholestatic liver disorders, hypokalemia, hypertonia, malaria, tuberculosis, abscesses, food poisoning, diabetes insipidus, chronic fatigue syndrome (CFS), and contact dermatitis. In combination with *Panax ginseng* and *Bupleurum falcatum*, licorice is used orally to help stimulate adrenal gland function, particularly in patients with a history of long-term corticosteroid use. As a component of the herbal formula Shakuyaku-kanzo-to, licorice is used to increase fertility in women with polycystic ovary syndrome. In combination with other herbs, licorice is used to treat prostate cancer and atopic dermatitis (eczema). Externally, licorice is used as a shampoo to reduce sebum secretion. Licorice is used as a flavoring in foods, beverages, and tobacco.[12]

Lobelia
Lobelia Inflata

This is an annual. The flowering parts and seeds are used medicinally. Carefully dust soil with tiny seed and press soil firmly. Keep wet until seed germinates, which may take one to three weeks. Water gently so as not to move seed. Internally, lobelia is taken for asthma, bronchitis, whooping cough, inducing sweating, and as a sedative. Lobelia is also used as an ingredient in smoking-cessation products and for treating apnea in newborn infants. Externally, lobelia is used for muscle inflammation, rheumatic nodules, bruises, sprains, insect bites, poison ivy, and ringworm. In manufacturing, lobelia is used in cough preparations and counterirritant products.[13]

Ma Huang
Ephedra sinica; Ephedra distachya

This herb prefers dry soil. The young stems and branchlets are the parts used medicinally. Plant in spring in cactus-mix potting soil, watering once a day and keeping warm. It sprouts in one to three weeks. Transplant to dry, fast-draining garden soil after a year in a pot. Internally, ephedra is taken for weight loss, obesity, enhanced athletic performance, nasal allergies and congestion; respiratory bronchospasm, asthma, bronchitis, colds, flu, swine flu, fever, chills, headache, anhidrosis, joint and bone pain, and as a diuretic for edema.[14]

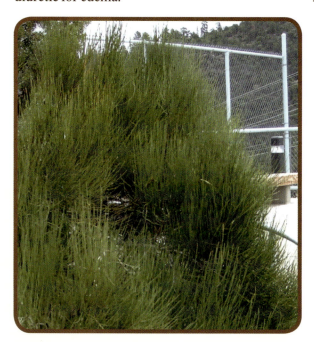

Brigham Tea, also called Mormon Tea, can grow huge in the wild. Brigham Tea is a natural source of ephedra.

Mormon Tea
Ephedra nevadensis

This is an evergreen desert plant. It prefers dry soil without fertile soil, and it grows in waste places, sand, and gravel. Green stemlike leaves that are black inside are used medicinally. Barely cover the seed, and keep it very warm, in light and moisture until germination. Grow in a pot for at least a year before transplanting. Over time, this plant becomes very large and is very long-lived. Reed-like stems are used to make tea. This seed is very hard to come by. Internally, Mormon tea is used for syphilis, gonorrhea, colds, kidney disorders, and as a "spring" tonic. Mormon tea is consumed as a beverage.[15]

Mullein (Common)
Verbascum thapsus, Verbascum densiflorum

This is a biennial medicinal herb. Press seed onto soil in spring or autumn and keep moist until germination, which takes one to two weeks. It grows up to three feet tall at the flowering stage. Its leaves are harvested to make a tincture to ease breathing, coughs, asthma, and colds, and also as a mild pain relief. It can be a reliable self-seeder. Mullein is taken by mouth for respiratory tract membrane inflammation, cough, whooping cough, tuberculosis, bronchitis, hoarseness, pneumonia, earache, colds, chills, flu, swine flu, fever, allergies, tonsillitis, tracheitis, asthma, diarrhea, colic, gastrointestinal bleeding, migraines, and gout. It is used as a sedative, narcotic, diuretic, and antirheumatic. The root is used for croup. Mullein is used externally for wounds, burns, hemorrhoids, bruises, frostbite, erysipelas, and inflamed mucosa. The leaves are used topically to soften and protect the skin. In manufacturing, mullein is used as a flavoring component in alcoholic beverages.[16]

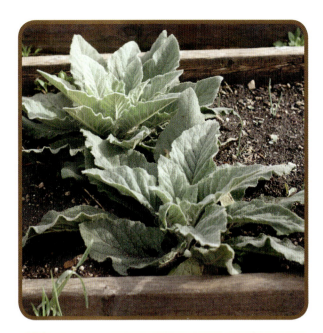

Mullein from the author's garden

Oregano
Origanum vulgare

This ancient herb is both medicinal and culinary. The stems, leaves, and flowers are used medicinally.

True oregano is taken for respiratory tract infections including influenza, common cold virus, croup, cough, asthma, bronchitis, indigestion, bloating, dysmenorrhea, rheumatoid arthritis, urinary tract infections (UTIs), headaches, heart conditions, intestinal parasites, allergies, sinusitis, arthritis, cold and flu, swine flu, earaches, and fatigue. Externally, oregano oil is used for acne, athlete's foot, dandruff, insect and spider bites, canker sores, gum disease, toothaches, psoriasis, seborrhea, ringworm, rosacea, muscle pain, varicose veins, warts, and as insect repellent. In foods and beverages, oregano is used as a culinary spice and a food preservative.[17]

Peppermint
Mentha Piperita

The leaves are the part used medicinally. Excellent for headaches, flavoring, homemade tooth powder, and relief of upset stomach. Creeping perennial (comes back year after year). Press seed into soil and keep moist until germination, which takes one to two weeks. Harvest when in bloom. Peppermint is taken for the common cold, cough, inflammation of the mouth and pharynx, sinusitis, fever, liver and gallbladder complaints, irritable bowel syndrome (IBS), cramps of the upper gastrointestinal (GI) tract and bile ducts, spasm associated with endoscopy procedures, dyspepsia, fever, flatulence, tension headache, nausea, vomiting, morning sickness, respiratory infections, dysmenorrhea, diarrhea, small intestinal bacterial overgrowth, and as a stimulant. Externally, peppermint oil is used for headache, myalgias, neuralgias, toothache, oral mucosa inflammation, rheumatic conditions, pruritus, urticaria,

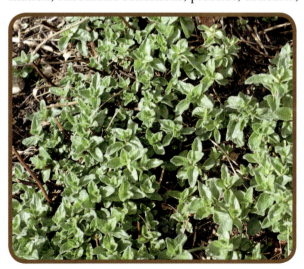

Oregano is used in both medicinal and culinary settings.

bacterial and viral infections, as an antispasmodic in barium enemas, and for repelling mosquitoes. As an inhalant, peppermint oil is used as an aromatic, for symptomatic treatment of cough and colds, and as an analgesic for pain. In foods and beverages, peppermint is a common flavoring agent. In manufacturing, peppermint oil is used as a fragrance component in soaps and cosmetics, and as a flavoring agent in pharmaceuticals.[18]

Plantain (Common or Great Plantain)
(Plantago major)

The roots, leaves, and flowers are used medicinally, but the leaves are used most often. It is a perennial medicinal herb. Plant in early spring in garden or pots. Barely cover seed, press soil firmly, and keep wet until germination, which can take six weeks. Used to make poultices for bites, stings, swelling, and irritated skin. It is an excellent self-seeder. Great Plantain has been used for cystitis with hematuria,

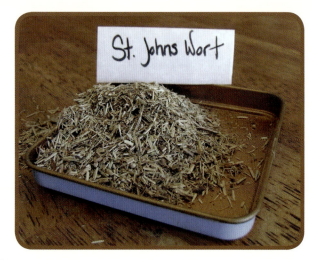

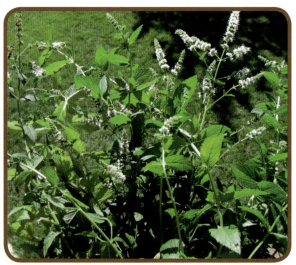

Peppermint leaves are excellent for headaches, flavoring, homemade tooth powder, and relief of upset stomach.

bronchitis, colds, and irritated or bleeding hemorrhoids, and as an antiseptic, anti-inflammatory, and antibacterial. Externally, plantain is used for dermatological conditions and eye irritation or discomfort.[19]

St. John's Wort
Hypericum perforatum

Flowering stems and flowers are the parts used medicinally. It prefers full sun. Plant in the spring. Press seeds into soil and keep it moist until germination, which takes about a week. This herb flowers in the second year. St. John's wort is taken internally for depression, dysthymia, anxiety, heart palpitations, mood swings caused by menopause, attention deficit-hyperactivity disorder (ADHD), obsessive-compulsive disorder (OCD), seasonal affective disorder (SAD), exhaustion, smoking cessation, fibromyalgia, chronic fatigue syndrome (CFS), menopause, fibrositis, headache, migraines, muscle pain, neuralgia, sciatica, cancer, vitiligo, HIV/AIDS, hepatitis C, weight loss, as a diuretic, and for irritable bowel syndrome (IBS). It is also taken by mouth to treat the symptoms of depression, including fatigue, loss of appetite, insomnia, and anxiety. Externally, oily St. John's wort preparations are used for treating bruises and abrasions, inflammation and muscle pain, first-degree burns, wound healing, bug bites, hemorrhoids, vitiligo, and neuralgia. In manufacturing, the hypericin-free extracts of St. John's wort are used in the making of alcoholic beverages.[20]

Self-Heal
Prunella vulgaris

Its leaves and stems are used in tea for internal and external wound healing and sore throats. It is a creeping evergreen ground cover herb. It will grow in either sun or shade. Self-Heal is taken internally for Crohn's disease, ulcerative colitis, HIV/AIDS, fever, headache, colic, vertigo, liver disease, spasm, diarrhea, and gastroenteritis; used as an antiseptic, expectorant, and astringent; and for mouth and throat ulcers, sore throat, and internal hemorrhaging. Externally it is also used for leukorrhea, gynecological disorders, wounds, and bruises.[21]

Soapwort (used for making homemade soap)
Saponaria officinalis

Perennial and very cold-hardy. Very old herb that has been used to make soap since before the time of Christ. Flowers, roots, stems, and leaves are used to make liquid soap. It has beautiful pink and white flowers. This herb likes sun to part-shade. It also likes moist soil. Barely cover the seed and keep it warm until germination. It grows two- to three-feet tall in full flower. Soapwort will spread if given regular water, so you may want to plant in pots or inside a border. It is taken internally for inflammation of mucous membranes in the upper and lower respiratory tract. Externally, soapwort is used as a remedy for poison ivy, acne, psoriasis, eczema, and boils. In manufacturing, soapwort is used as an ingredient in soaps, herbal shampoos, and detergents. It is used as a foaming agent in beer.[22]

Spearmint
Mentha spicata

This is a perennial. It is used as an ingredient in homemade toothpaste and drinks, teas, and compresses. It likes moist, rich soil in sun or shade. Press into soil and keep moist until germination, which takes about a week. Water only gently, so as not to dislodge germinating roots. Will spread to form a patch if given regular water, so keep in pots or inside a border for control. Spearmint is taken internally for flatulence, indigestion, nausea, sore throat, diarrhea, colds, headaches, toothaches, cramps, cancer, bile duct and gallbladder inflammation, gallstones, upper gastrointestinal tract spasms, irritable bowel syndrome (IBS), and inflammation of respiratory tract. It is also used as an aromatic, stimulant, antiseptic, local anesthetic, and antispasmodic. Externally, spearmint is used for oral mucosal inflammation, arthritis, local muscle and nerve pain, and skin conditions including pruritus and urticaria. In foods and beverages, spearmint is used as a flavoring agent. In manufacturing, spearmint is used in health food

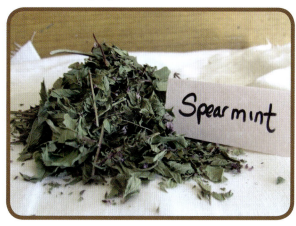

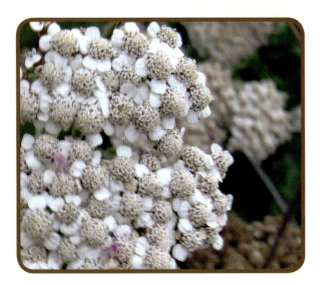

Fresh yarrow leaves are chewed to relieve toothache.

products, cosmetics, and oral hygiene products such as mouthwash and toothpaste.[23]

Stevia
Stevia rebaudiana

Stevia is a green leafy herb that is sweeter than sugar but does not contain any sugar at all and does not spike the glycemic index. Some studies have shown it lowers high blood pressure but does not lower normal blood pressure. Start indoors in early spring. Soil must remain evenly moist for germination. Press seed to soil surface. Stevia takes two to four weeks to germinate, and has sixty to seventy percent germination. Young plants must be kept moist. Transfer it outside after the last frost. Stevia will not thrive in hot summer weather but will suddenly grow rapidly in the fall. Cut plants to about two inches tall and dry the leaves for kitchen use. Bring the plant indoors to overwinter on a sunny windowsill, and this plant will be perennial. Medicinally, stevia is taken internally as a weight loss aid; for treating diabetes; for contraception, hypertension, heartburn, and lowering uric acid levels; and as a cardiotonic and diuretic. In foods, stevia is used as a non-caloric sweetener and flavor enhancer.[24]

Valerian
Valeriana officinalis

This is a perennial. The roots are the part used medicinally. It likes sun to part-shade. Start indoors in the spring. Seeds must have light to germinate, so only press them onto soil. Germination is slow—two weeks or more. Baby plants look nothing like mature plants. It likes well-drained soil with frequent watering. Valerian is taken by mouth for insomnia, dyssomnia, anxiety-related restlessness, sleeping disorders, depression, infantile convulsions, mild tremors, epilepsy, attention-deficit hyperactivity disorder (ADHD), chronic fatigue syndrome (CFS), muscle and joint pain, anxiety nervous asthma, hysterical states, hypochondria, headaches, migraine, indigestion, menstrual cramps, and hot flashes. Externally, valerian is used as a bath additive for restlessness and sleep disorders. In manufacturing, the extracts and essential oil are used as flavoring in foods and beverages.[25]

Yarrow
Achillea millefolium

Yarrow is an herb used in tea and cough syrups for flu, sinus, colds, and asthma. It is a perennial. Stems, leaves, and flowers are used medicinally. Yarrow is a reliable self-seeder, but it does not spread vigorously, so you don't have to worry about it taking over. Yarrow is taken internally for fever, common cold, allergic rhinitis, amenorrhea, dysentery, diarrhea, loss of appetite, mild or spastic gastrointestinal (GI) tract discomfort; to induce sweating; and for thrombotic conditions with hypertension, including cerebral and coronary thromboses. The fresh leaves are chewed to relieve toothache. Externally, yarrow is used as a styptic; for bleeding hemorrhoids; for wounds; and as a sitz bath for painful, lower pelvic, cramp-like conditions of psychosomatic origin in women. In combination with other herbs, yarrow is used for bloating, flatulence, mild gastrointestinal (GI) cramping, and nervous gastrointestinal complaints. In foods, the young leaves and flowers of yarrow are used in salads. In manufacturing, yarrow is also used as a cosmetic cleanser and in snuff. Yarrow oil is used in shampoos.[26]

WHEN TO PICK HERBS

It is best to pick herbs in the late morning, for two reasons. First, plants should be free of morning dew when you harvest them because you don't want additional moisture on the plants. Early morning is not a good time to harvest fresh herbs because of lingering dew. Second, the heat of day can wilt herbs, making them less than their prime. Just as you pick garden vegetables at their prime and not when they are wilted, herbs are also best before they have suffered the heat of the day. Late morning is the time when the dew has gone but the sun has not had time to wilt the plants.

Leafy herbs are often at their medicinal prime in late spring. Bark is generally at its medicinal prime when the sap is running in late spring or summer. Roots are at their medicinal prime in autumn after the plant's summer cycle has ended and the roots are gathering strength for winter. Roots are also at their lowest moisture content in the autumn, which is ideal for drying roots for later use.

HOW TO DRY HERBS

Medicinal herbs should be air-dried outside of direct sunlight. Direct sunlight should be avoided because it can trans-evaporate the oils in the herbs along with the water, which will damage the medicinal quality of the herbs. While they are drying, herbs should be kept in a place where bugs cannot get to them, and where they will be free of debris floating in the air, such as pet hair or household dust. Herbs are dry enough for storage if they crinkle when handled and do not feel cold to the touch. The cold would indicate the presence of moisture.

Whether you are harvesting roots, leaves and stems, or flowers, all parts should be perfectly clean and then dried in the open air. Mesh-enclosed herb drying racks sell on Amazon and other online retailers for about thirty dollars. These drying racks have a large capacity and keep out bugs and other potential contaminants. Simply pick your herbs at the peak of health and then rinse them with clean, cold water. The herbs can be cut into six-inch lengths to better fit into the drying rack, and then spun dry in a salad spinner. If you don't have a salad spinner, you can pat the herbs in a clean cotton cloth. Place them in the dryer and hang the dryer in a room-temperature place away from direct sunlight.

Air drying allows moisture to evaporate from the herbs slowly, while retaining their essential oils and other volatile compounds. If you try to use a heat source to dry the herbs faster, you are likely to damage their medicinal qualities.

Storing Dried Herbs

Dried herbs can be kept in a common cupboard in clear glass jars covered by lids to keep out

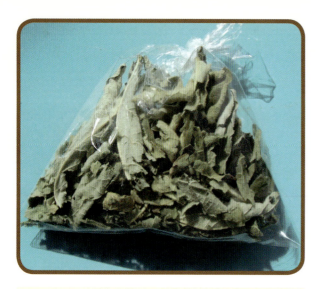

Dried mullein for tincturing.

contaminants. Dried herbs will last several years, though you may need to increase the herbal dosage with older herbs as they slowly lose their potency.

FINDING HELP

If you are new to herbal medicine, you will quickly be astonished how many people around you are using herbs medicinally. Experienced herbalists are almost always happy to help a newcomer. There is untold value in seeking out people in your local area who have experience and wisdom to share with you. They will know what herbs grow best where you are and where the wild herbs might be found, and they can share with you their favorite recipes, remedies, and experiences with herbs.

This book, aimed at beginners, has not even skimmed the surface of the world of medicinal herbs. While we have attempted to include as much basic information as possible, you will quickly learn that there are myriad other herbs, recipes, remedies,

salves, preparations, decoctions, and methods that are not touched on in this book. The more you research, the more the world of natural medicine will open up to you—and no one is a better teacher than a friend or neighbor in your area who can share with you their own personal experiences, recipes, and wisdom. Don't be surprised if you stumble upon a community of like-minded people who will be happy to divide their plants with you, recommend favorite stores or sources, and give you samples of their remedies and salves to try for yourself. As you learn more, these people will become a source of information as you encounter new situations that you want to confront with herbal healing options. They will be able to answer your questions and guide you according to their own hard-won experience. If you are not sure where to begin looking for these people, here are some suggestions:

Your family

Begin by asking around your family whether anyone has experience with specific herbs or tinctures. Many times you will be surprised to learn who is a secret herbal practitioner! Along the way, be sure to write down as many of the remedies and recipes in your family as you can. One great problem with the wisdom of natural healing is that in many cases it was handed down orally and never written down— and then the world began to tilt toward modern medicine, and today, finding out exactly what your grandmother's mother used in that poultice decades ago can be frustratingly difficult. While many families and communities have recorded stories about a local doctor or herbal healer who was the stuff of legend, the recipes and specifics have almost never been written down and, unfortunately, neither have the stories. We need to collect as much information as possible about what remains before it is lost. If you have herbal knowledge that you wish to share, please email calebwarnock@yahoo.com and share your stories, recipes, or any other relevant information. Caleb may share your information on his blog at CalebWarnock.blogspot.com.

Local Herb and Health Food Stores

Perhaps the fastest way in the world to get "plugged in" to the alternative medicine community is to walk into your local health food store and simply ask the staff if they know of any local groups, experts, or classes. The answer is almost always a resounding yes. And if the answer is no, then here is a surefire way to find the "in" crowd—just hang out on the herb and tincture aisle and see who is browsing and buying. Introduce yourself as someone new to herbal health and healing in the area, and ask them if they know of anyone who is a great resource.

Online Communities

If you go to Facebook and type "medicinal herbs" into the search bar, you will be introduced to a whole new world of friends and communities who celebrate natural healing, medicinal herbs, historical herbal books, and much, much more. You will find many diverse groups—people specializing in roots, books, edible wild plants, seeds, and more. And this is just on Facebook. A Google search for any medicinal herb topic—the name of an herb or a tincture, the name of an herbal book—will lead you to volumes of information. We have included some of the best websites for "jumping off" the diving board into the online pool of information in the Resources chapter at the end of this book.

Notes

1. Anise," Natural Medicines Comprehensive Database, accessed October 21, 2014
2. "Astragalus," Natural Medicines Comprehensive Database, accessed October 21, 2014
3. "Black Cohosh," Natural Medicines Comprehensive Database, accessed October 21, 2014
4. "Calendula," Natural Medicines Comprehensive Database, accessed October 21, 2014
5. "Cayenne," Natural Medicines Comprehensive Database, accessed October 21, 2014
6. "Comfrey," Natural Medicines Comprehensive Database, accessed October 21, 2014
7. "Elecampane," Natural Medicines Comprehensive Database, accessed October 21, 2014
8. "Feverfew," Natural Medicines Comprehensive Database, accessed October 21, 2014
9. "German Chamomile," Natural Medicines Comprehensive Database, accessed October 21, 2014
10. "White Horehound," Natural Medicines Comprehensive Database, accessed October 21, 2014,
11. "Hyssop," Natural Medicines Comprehensive Database, accessed October 21, 2014
12. "Licorice," Natural Medicines Comprehensive Database, accessed October 21, 2014
13. "Lobelia," Natural Medicines Comprehensive Database, accessed October 21, 2014
14. "Ma Huang," Natural Medicines Comprehensive Database, accessed October 21, 2014
15. "Mormon Tea," Natural Medicines Comprehensive Database, accessed October 21, 2014
16. "Mullein," Natural Medicines Comprehensive Database, accessed October 21, 2014
17. "Oregano," Natural Medicines Comprehensive Database, accessed October 21, 2014
18. "Peppermint," Natural Medicines Comprehensive Database, accessed October 21, 2014
19. "Plantain," Natural Medicines Comprehensive Database, accessed October 21, 2014
20. "St. John's Wort," Natural Medicines Comprehensive Database, accessed October 21, 2014

21. "Self-Heal," Natural Medicines Comprehensive Database, accessed October 21, 2014

22. "Soapwort," Natural Medicines Comprehensive Database, accessed October 21, 2014

23. "Spearmint," Natural Medicines Comprehensive Database, accessed October 21, 2014

24. "Stevia," Natural Medicines Comprehensive Database, accessed October 21, 2014

25. "Valerian," Natural Medicines Comprehensive Database, accessed October 21, 2014

26. "Yarrow," Natural Medicines Comprehensive Database, accessed October 21, 2014

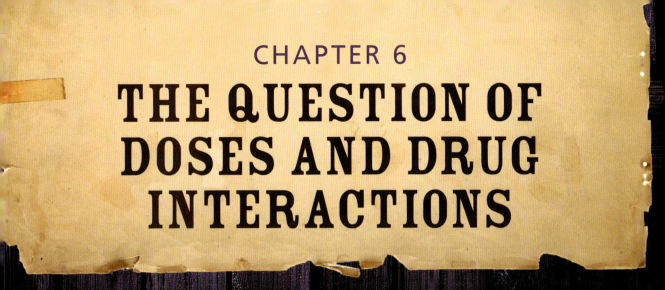

CHAPTER 6

THE QUESTION OF DOSES AND DRUG INTERACTIONS

Before we go any further in this book, we need to talk about an important difference between herbal remedies and prescription drugs. One of the challenges for people who are new to herbal medicine is the question of how to know what the correct "dose" of an herbal remedy is.

The question of proper dosage is made easier when you think about herbal medicine as being based in food, not chemicals. Our modern prescription drugs are often based on laboratory chemicals that are so powerful they are dangerous in the wrong doses. In fact, they are often dangerous even at the "correct" doses, as indicated by the long list of side effects that accompanies most prescription drugs.

Medicinal herbs are different. Herbs are food.

In this book, we will ask you to look at garlic as not only a food, but an antibiotic. Onions become pharmaceutical. Apple cider vinegar becomes serum. These are each food, but in this book, we will show you how and why to use them as medicine. The same is true of backyard herbs—horehound, cayenne peppers, lemon balm, and hyssop, just to name a few. We will encourage you to grow your own when possible, or buy them if need be.

Everything in this book is natural—even the tincture solutions. Vinegar was made at home for thousands of years. Vegetable glycerin is a natural byproduct of extracting oil from vegetables. Ethyl alcohol is the natural byproduct of yeast. The foods-as-medicine that we recommend are natural, and the herbs are natural. So it should be no surprise that the "doses" of these medicines are "natural" too. By natural, we mean they are intuitive, often based on personal experience instead of clinical trials.

Many herbal enthusiasts would love it if the medical community would run clinical trials on herbs. But they are not interested. Not at all. Why? Because herbs cannot be patented or "owned" by a corporation. Since they cannot be proprietary, there is no profit in them, so they are ignored by medical corporations that must, by law, make money for their stockholders. These companies invest only in drugs they can create in laboratories and thus legally own—they are betting not on your health, but on a windfall of cash if they win government approval.

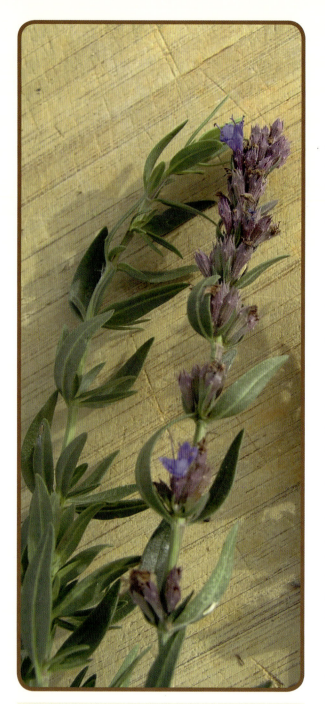

Hyssop in flower in Caleb Warnock's backyard.

(Government approval, as we have seen in many cases, does not always mean a drug is safe.)

Though herbs like valerian and nettle have been used for hundreds of years, we have no modern information about what the ideal scientific "dose" of these medications should be, because there is not a company in the world willing to invest the cash to do clinical studies—after all, a single clinical study can cost $100 million, and determining dosages and scientific "validity" requires a series of ever-larger clinical studies by law.[1]

But don't mistake a lack of clinical studies for a lack of proof that medicinal herbs work. We have hundreds of years of information—even modern information—showing they work. But when it comes to figuring out a dose, we can only rely on the experience of those who have used these herbs for decades.

Here are some general guidelines for deciding what dosage is right for you and your family.

1. *Start small.* Herbal doses are traditionally small and conservative. For example, in this book we recommend that when you are making an herbal tea, you use one teaspoon of dried herb to one cup of water. Why? Because this recipe works for us, and has worked for untold numbers of herbal home practitioners. If you have never swallowed a tincture of cayenne pepper before, you would be wise to start with a single drop. Catnip tea, on the other hand, is much more mild and it is reasonable to think that a teaspoon sieved in a cup of hot water is a good place to start.

2. *Know your own allergies.* If you know you are one of the rare people in the world who have an allergy to the mint family of plants, then you should not use peppermint, spearmint, borage, catnip, lemon balm (often called melissa), or other medicinal herbs in the mint family. Before you take any herb, make sure the

plant is not in a family of plants that you know you are allergic to.

3. *Avoid hypochondria*. This can be a real concern, especially to people who are brand new to herbal medicine. Caleb taught a class once about how he uses pine sap (crude turpentine) as an immune stimulant. During the class, Caleb and the students went on an herbal walk to nearby pine trees, where Caleb showed them what pine sap looks like and how to harvest it without damaging the tree. Later, some of the students drove to Caleb's house to tour his geothermal greenhouse. During the tour, one student, full of concern, told Caleb that he had eaten one drop of pine sap (Caleb's recommended dose) and was now experiencing a back ache. The student was concerned this meant he was having a reaction to the pine sap. After explaining that one drop of pine sap is unlikely to have the power to cause a backache in anyone, Caleb offered a different diagnosis.

"Perhaps it could be sitting in a hard chair for seven hours of classes today that could have caused your back pain," Caleb said.

"Oh, I guess so," said the student, clearly relieved that he wasn't dying of some kind of mythical pine sap poisoning.

Hypochondria is real. Having anxiety about your health—especially when it comes to trying remedies that are new to you—is entirely normal. It helps to keep this in mind—does it make more sense to have anxiety about a teaspoon of lemon balm, which has been used for a thousand years, or a prescription drug, which comes with its own long list of known side effects?

4. *Use caution*. While choosing an herbal dosage for an adult might require some experimenting and some faith in the advice of experienced herbal practitioners, finding a dose for a young child or pregnant woman must be left to experts. We suggest you find a medical doctor who is also experienced in herbal remedies to consult before using any herbal remedy if you are pregnant, or before giving any dose to a child under the age of two years old. When dealing with young children and pregnant women, an abundance of caution is wise.

THE PROBLEM OF MODERN DRUG INTERACTIONS

As mentioned earlier in this book, herbal medicine has been successfully practiced for millennia and without it most of us would not be here today. But within the past few decades, the world of medicine has changed in an unprecedented way with the invention of prescription drugs created from non-natural chemicals made to exist only because of complicated, multi-million-dollar laboratories. These drugs save lives, and they are powerful.

Herbs are powerful too. But the problem of prescription drugs and herbs negatively interacting is not a conundrum any of our ancestor-practitioners ever had to worry about.

At the outset, we should say that the problem is not just limited to herbal medicines. It is generally well known by now that certain citrus fruits, especially grapefruit, can wreak havoc on the effects of certain prescription medications—85 different drugs, if the Internet is to be believed. There are also other non-herb foods that "tamper" with modern drugs, either quashing or dangerously magnifying their medicinal powers. So it should not shock anyone to know that medicinal herbs can mess with the outcome of pharmacy drugs.

Ironically, warnings from drug companies and health officials about the potential for herbs to interact with pharmaceuticals are some of the primary scientific evidence offered by doctors that medicinal herbs not only work but are powerful in their own right. Many ancient herbs have the potential to conflict with prescription and over-the-counter medications. Lobelia, calendula, skullcap, and St. John's Wort, to name four examples, are known to interact with some medications. Because of this, we as consumers have an obligation to think differently about herbal medicine than any of the generations who came before us. Herbs were a normal part of everyday life for them—laboratory-crafted chemicals and drugs were not.

It boils down to this: If you are taking any prescription or over-the counter pharmaceutical, never take herbal remedies of any kind without first consulting a medical doctor who is experienced in alternative medicine. The interactions between herbs and modern drugs can be dangerous, even fatal. Some herbs can potentially make a prescription drug ineffective. Others can heighten or even greatly multiply the effect of modern pharmaceuticals.

The conflict between modern and ancient remedies is even more dangerous when we are dosing our friends and neighbors. Once, during an herbal medicine class that Kirsten taught around Caleb's kitchen table, a woman volunteered the information that she had been secretly giving her husband an herbal medication by mixing it in his food without his knowledge. This is exactly the kind of dangerous "helpfulness" that can give herbal medicine a bad name. While an herbal decoction may work wonders for Caleb or Kirsten, the same medicine may have an entirely different result on someone else who is taking a daily handful of pharmaceuticals and is in poor health.

It is always exciting when an herbal remedy works—you naturally want to tell other people about

it. But while we tell our friends and neighbors that skullcap helped us overcome our sleeplessness, we may not know that those friends are already taking powerful prescription sleeping aids that may go haywire when combined with skullcap. We cannot overemphasize that if someone is taking a modern drug, research, in consultation with a medical doctor experienced in practicing herbal medicine, is required.

Any attempt in this book to give you specific information about potential interactions would likely be outdated even before this book hits shelves, because new drugs are introduced regularly. But there are places you can go to get up-to-date information for your own research. Here is a list of places where you can do your own research about the potential interactions between herbs and pharmaceuticals (courtesy of SeedRenaissance.com):

• The U.S. National Institutes of Health's "Herbs At A Glance" service is perhaps the premier place to find the history of medicinal herbs, uses, known drug interactions, and information about modern scientific studies. No one should take any medicinal herb without consulting the information and warnings available here.[2]

• The Natural Medicines Comprehensive Database offers "Unbiased, Scientific Clinical Information on Complementary, Alternative, and Integrative Therapies" and is operated by the Therapeutic Research Center, which is funded by pharmacists, pharmacy technicians and others who pay for subscriptions. The information they provide is vast and fascinating. They offer drug interaction warnings, effectiveness ratings, information on clinical studies, a searchable database about how specific herbs interact with specific diseases, and more.[3]

- MedlinePlus is a service of the U.S. National Library of Medicine, and provides a guide to herbs and supplements, including informtion about potential drug interactions.[4]

- Webmd.com/vitamins-supplements/default.aspx—This website includes a list of the potential interactions and side effects of medicinal herbs.[5]

- Umm.edu/health/medical/altmed—The University of Maryland Medical Center's Complementary and Alternative Medicine Guide, which includes a list of the potential interactions and side effects of medicinal herbs.[6]

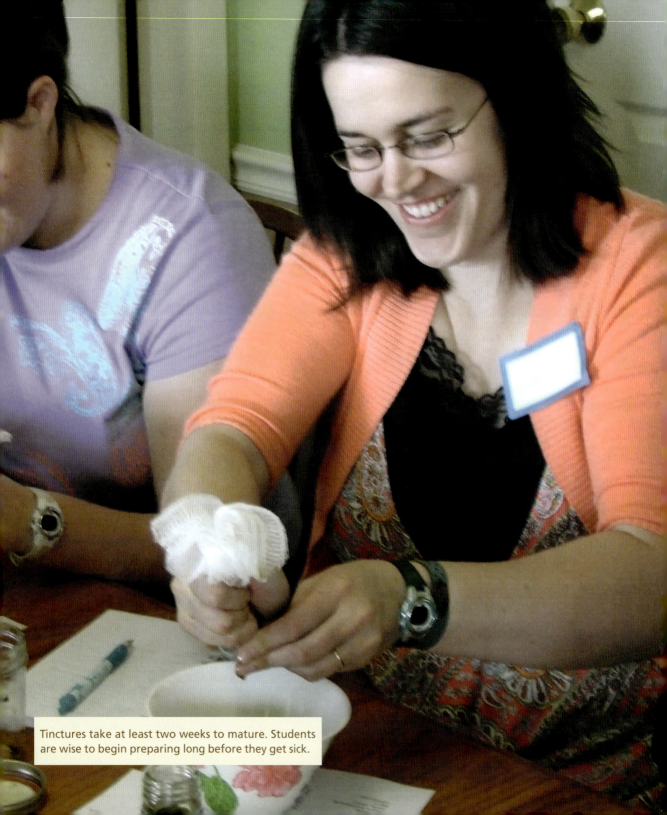

Tinctures take at least two weeks to mature. Students are wise to begin preparing long before they get sick.

CHAPTER 7
TINCTURES FOR BEGINNERS

A tincture is a liquid, mixed with herbs, to create herbal medicine. Tinctures have a long history of use, and continue to be popular to this day. You, the reader, almost certainly have several tinctures in your home right now. Vanilla extract, used in baking and cooking, is one of the most common. All of the different cough syrups available at the pharmacy or grocery store are also a form of tincture. Any flavor extract that you might buy at the store for candy making or baking is a tincture. Tincture of iodine used to be in nearly every house in America, for treating basic cuts and scrapes (remember how it used to sting!)

Simply put, a tincture is a method for preserving the medicine that occurs naturally in certain herbs.

In this book, we will introduce you to the three basic methods for making a tincture at home. No matter which tincture method you choose, they all have something in common—they use a liquid to extract the medicinal (and sometimes culinary) qualities out of the herbs, and preserve those qualities for later use.

About 60 A.D., a Roman physician-pharmacist named Pedanius Dioscorides wrote five volumes of a book that today we call *De Materia Medica* ("Of Medical Materials"). This book lists the medicinal herbs of his day and their uses. *De Materia Medica* has never been out of print in nearly two millenia. The book has been immensely popular and nearly globally used for centuries. In it, Dioscorides talks about soaking certain herbs—lemon balm, for example—in wine and then drinking the wine as medicine. This is a very early use of medicinal tinctures. Hyssop used in medicinal tea is a favorite backyard herb, and it is fascinating to be able to use the same herb, for the same medical purpose, as practiced by Dioscorides nearly 2,000 years ago. As an example of the long history of medicinal tinctures, here is Dioscorides' recipe for a tincture of hyssop (note: "must" is pressed grapes with the skin and seeds):

"Put one pound of bruised hyssop leaves (wrapped in a thin linen cloth) into nine gallons of must and also put in small stones so that the bundle subsides to the bottom. After forty days strain it and put it in another jar. It is good for disorders in the chest, side, and lungs, and for old coughs, and asthma. It is diuretic, good for griping, and the periodical chills of fevers, and it induces the menstrual flow."[1]

Medicinal tinctures for internal use must be made with one of three natural solvents—ethyl alcohol (typically vodka), glycerin, or vinegar. These three "solvents" have the ability to dissolve and preserve the specific medicinal molecules that are naturally produced in certain herbs.

Medicinal herbs have been traced back 5,000 years, starting with the Sumerians and the Chinese. Hippocrates was an herbalist who authored the statement "First do no harm" that is cited today by medical doctors when they make their oath. Tinctures have the ability to withdraw the medicinal properties of plants and preserve them indefinitely. That is highly recommended so your efforts are not wasted. As we make tinctures, we do not always use all we make. Having them preserved and in storage is beneficial for emergencies and saves money and time.

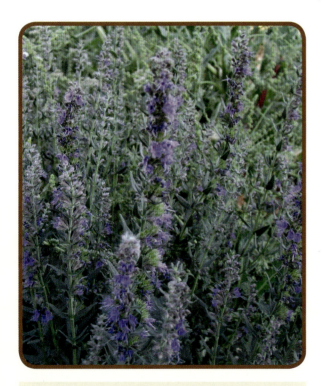

In manufacturing, hyssop oil is used as a fragrance in soaps and cosmetics.

TYPE OF HERBS USED IN TINCTURE

When making tinctures, using dry herbs is best, but there are a few herbs that are sold commercially only in powder form, such as cayenne. When using a powdered herb, it is more difficult to separate the tincture from the herb, but of course it is worth the extra work. There are also herbs that are in a resin form, like pine sap and myrrh. These herbs need to be made in an alcohol tincture and are usually quite powerful. Pine sap is a natural antiseptic and can act as a band-aid as well. Myrrh is Kirsten's favorite herb for fighting bacteria and fungus, and you can read more about it the Remedies chapter of this book.

Ideally, dried medicinal herbs should be used within two years. If your dried herb is more than two years old, keep two rules in mind: First, if the herb still has a scent, it still has some medicinal properties. Second, the older the herb is, the more of it you will need to use to get the same effect as dried herbs that are fresh.

CREATING A TINCTURE OF ETHYL ALCOHOL

This is more commonly called an alcohol tincture or vodka tincture. Before going any further, we want to point out that neither of us—Kirsten nor Caleb—drink alcohol. We are both members of The Church of Jesus Christ of Latter-day Saints (the Mormons), and we choose not to drink alcohol. You can easily remove the alcohol of any vodka tincture you make at home, and this book will explain how. We will also point out that you, the reader, use alcohol tinctures routinely in your home in the form of cough syrups from the grocery store. Alcohol has a long and

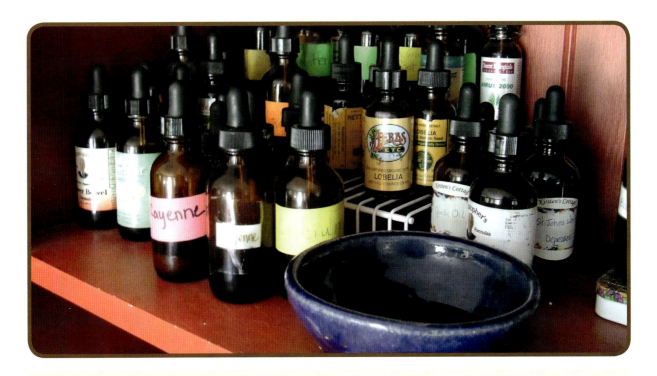

A chest full of herbs and tinctures like the one pictured above will become a family heirloom.

important history of medical use exactly because of its ability to "solve" or extract and perfectly preserve medicine from herbs.

If there is a person who is an alcoholic, it would be best to use only the glycerin tinctures. As you will see below, all alcohol tinctures can be made into glycerin tinctures by the use of heat and patience. Most children would prefer the sweet taste of a glycerin tincture. And getting them to take their medicine is a large part of healing. Just ask Mary Poppins.

Ethyl alcohol (vodka) is excellent for making tinctures for several reasons:

1. Ethyl alcohol is a perfect preservative, and tinctures made with this method can last for years.

2. Ethyl alcohol is the most powerful solution of the three tincture choices. Some medicinal herbs, such as mullein, simply do not release their medicine easily when tinctured in glycerin or vinegar, but are easily "solved" by ethyl alcohol.

3. Ethyl alcohol is a strong solvent for both acid and alkaline herbs.

RECIPE FOR TINCTURE OF ETHYL ALCOHOL

- 1 ounce of dried medicinal herb (example: mullein)

- 4 ounces of good-quality 100-proof vodka

STEP 1. Use only good-quality dried herbs for making tincture. Make sure the herbs have not been sprayed with pesticides or other chemicals. Place dried herbs in a clean glass jar. Pour vodka over the herbs.

STEP 2. Seal the jar with a tight lid and store in a dry, dark place for at least two weeks. Shake the jar every day or as often as you walk by.

STEP 3. Label your tincture immediately—don't wait. The tincture will begin to darken and the herbs will begin to "melt," for lack of a better word. You might be tempted to think you will remember what is in the tincture, or that you will be able to recognize the herbs in the jar, but tinctures are medicine and you should not rely on memory. Never use an unlabeled tincture.

STEP 4. After two weeks, use cheesecloth (a loosely woven cotton that can be purchased at most grocery stores) or a reusable, machine-washable muslin or polyester bag (available at SeedRenaissance.com; click on "apothecary") to strain the liquid, removing the herb. When a tincture has matured, it is essential to remove the spent herbs from the liquid. There are two ways to do this:

Kirsten's Method

STEP 1. Shake your mature tincture. Place a strainer (a pasta strainer is fine) into a bowl. Place your cheesecloth or reusable bag into the strainer. This elevates the material, allowing it to drip into the bowl. Pour the mature tincture into your straining cloth or bag.

STEP 2. Using your hands, squeeze the herbs in the cloth to get out the last of the liquid. If you are using cheesecloth, it can be discarded.

STEP 3. Open a sanitized glass jar and pour the tincture into the jar to store.

Caleb's Method

STEP 1. A potato ricer is a funny-looking gadget once widely used to mash potatoes. It resembles an old-fashioned pump handle. You can find them in kitchen stores, or in almost any antique store. Place a potato ricer in a bowl. Line the ricer with cheesecloth that has been folded into thirds, or place your reusable bag inside the ricer. Shake your mature tincture. Pour it into the cheesecloth or reusable bag. The tincture liquid will strain through the cheesecloth into the bowl, leaving the spent herbs in the cloth.

STEP 2. Using the handle of the ricer, squeeze the herbs in the cloth to get out the last of the liquid. Compost the spent herbs. If using cheesecloth, you can throw it away.

STEP 3. Open a sanitized glass jar and pour the tincture into the jar to store.

NOTE: Any mature tincture made with a fine powdery herb, such as cayenne, must be strained with muslin or a clean cotton kitchen cloth instead of cheesecloth. This is necessary to strain the fine powder from the liquid. Straining a powder with muslin or cotton toweling is a slower process than straining with cheesecloth, and you may need to strain small amounts at a time.

To remove the alcohol from a mature tincture

STEP 1. Once your tincture has matured, and you have strained it, you may remove the alcohol. To do this, bring the mature strained tincture to a boil on the stove in a stainless steel pan. You can remove the alcohol from as much or as little tincture as you want at one time. Vodka that is 100 proof is made of equal parts distilled water and pure alcohol, so when boiling reduces the tincture by half, the alcohol has been removed. Be cautious—the alcohol dissipates very fast—likely faster than you will expect. Remove the pan from the heat immediately after the volume of your liquid had reduced by half, because prolonged exposure to heat can damage or destroy the medicinal qualities you have extracted from the herbs.

STEP 2. Cool the remaining liquid and use within several weeks. A tincture with the alcohol removed should not be stored long-term, because the alcohol is the preservative, and once it is gone the medicine can begin to oxidize, age, and lose potency. For long-term storage of a tincture, keep the alcohol tincture intact and remove the alcohol only just before use. It is not necessary to remove the alcohol from the tincture, but it is recommended that the alcohol be removed before giving the tincture to children.

CREATING A TINCTURE OF VEGETABLE GLYCERIN

Vegetable glycerin is a by-product of extracting oil from certain vegetables. Vegetable glycerin is a clear, odorless syrup-like liquid that has a naturally sweet flavor. You can purchase it at any health food store or online.

Although it has nearly a third more calories per teaspoon than sugar, glycerin does not feed the bacteria that cause cavities. It is widely used in the U.S. in medicine, food, cosmetics, and soap.

While we recommend that you use vegetable glycerin, you can also buy glycerins that are a byproduct of the process of creating gasoline and oil. Petroleum-derived glycerin is 99.5% pure. However, that 0.5 percent impurity is made up of petrochemicals that can be damaging to human health. While vegetable glycerin may also have impurities as a result of the extraction process, those impurities are going to be vegetable based, making them safe for human consumption.

In chemistry terms, glycerin, also called glycerol, is a sugar-alcohol compound. A sugar alcohol compound is a molecular description only; glycerin is not a form of alcohol and does not have any of the effects of alcohol. It is not going to intoxicate you. Glycerin is safe for children. When chemists refer to glycerin as a sugar-alcohol compound, they are referring only to its chemical structure.

RECIPE FOR TINCTURE OF GLYCERIN

- 1 ounce of dried medicinal herb (example: yarrow)

- 2 ounces of vegetable glycerin

- 2 ounces of distilled water

- additional ½ ounce of distilled water (optional)

STEP 1. Mix the glycerin and distilled water, stirring to incorporate.

STEP 2. Use only good quality dried herbs for making

tincture. Make sure the herbs have not been sprayed with pesticides or other chemicals. Place dried herbs in a clean glass jar. Pour the mixture of glycerin and distilled water over the herbs. Seal the jar with a tight lid and store in a dry, dark place for at least two weeks. Shake the jar every day or whenever you pass by. If your preparation is too thick to shake, you can add the extra half-ounce of distilled water.

STEP 3. After at least two weeks, use cheesecloth or a reusable bag to strain the liquid, removing the herb. (For straining instructions, see the alcohol tincture recipe). Store the liquid in a jar of dark glass. Be sure to label the jar. Store in a dry, dark place.

STEP 4. Label your tincture immediately—don't wait. The tincture will begin to darken and the herbs will begin to "melt" for lack of a better word. You might be tempted to think you will remember what is in the tincture, or that you will be able to recognize the herbs in the jar, but tinctures are medicine and you should not rely on memory. Never use an unlabeled tincture.

RECIPE FOR TINCTURE OF VINEGAR

- 1 ounce of dried medicinal herb (example, lobelia)

- 4 ounces of good-quality white or apple cider vinegar

STEP 1. Use only good-quality dried herbs for making tinctures. Make sure the herbs have not been sprayed with pesticides or other chemicals. Place dried herbs in a clean glass jar. Pour vinegar over the herbs.

STEP 2. Seal the jar with a tight lid and store in a dry, dark place for at least two weeks. Shake the jar every day or as often as you pass by.

STEP 3. After two weeks, use a cheesecloth reusable bag to strain the liquid, removing the herb. (For straining instructions, see the alcohol tincture recipe.) Store the liquid in a jar of dark glass. Be sure to label the jar. Store in a dry, dark place.

STEP 4. Label your tincture immediately—don't wait. The tincture will begin to darken and the herbs will begin to "melt," for lack of a better word. You might be tempted to think you will remember what is in the tincture, or that you will be able to recognize the herbs in the jar, but tinctures are medicine and you should not rely on memory. Never use an unlabeled tincture.

HOW TO STORE A TINCTURE

There is a difference of opinion in the natural healing world about whether to expose a tincture to sunlight or not. Kirsten likes to put it on her windowsill while it is maturing with the herb in the liquid. Once the tincture has been strained, keep it in a dark place, or in a jar or bottle made of dark glass. Special brown glass or dark glass bottles for tincture storage can be purchased at most health food stores, herb stores, or online. A cupboard is NOT dark enough. You can also purchase or build a special herb cabinet for your home. This will become a family heirloom.

TINCTURE QUESTIONS AND ANSWERS

QUESTION: **Can I use fresh herbs, instead of dried herbs, for making a tincture?**

ANSWER: Our suggestion for making tinctures is to use the dried herb. The reason for this is moisture content. With dried herbs you can better determine how much of the herb will make the correct potency for your tincture, while moisture content in the herb can dilute the tincture. The amount of moisture in a plant will vary, which will make the effectiveness of your tincture unpredictable. The mathematical solution to determining the amount of moisture in a plant is complicated but can be done (for information, see *The Herbal Medicine Cabinet* by Debra St. Claire[2]). If you want your tinctures to be as potent as they are meant to be, without using the math, use the dried

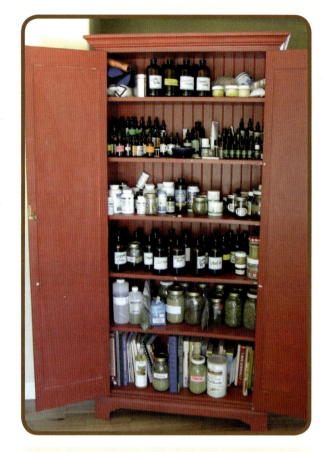

Kirsten Skirvin's home cabinet of herbal remedies.

herb. It will give you consistency and confidence in your herbs and their dosage.

QUESTION: **Can I use a less expensive vodka?**

ANSWER: When making an alcohol tincture, the vodka should be 100 proof (50 percent alcohol and 50 percent water). Some less expensive vodkas are 40 percent alcohol and 60 percent water. If you use a 40/60 vodka, your tincture may never mature. If you cannot find a good quality 100-proof vodka, you can buy Everclear, which is 200 proof (100 percent alcohol) and dilute it with distilled water. Use distilled water because it absorbs minerals.

QUESTION: Can I combine tinctures?

ANSWER: Yes. Tinctures should be created individually—one herb per tincture. But once your tinctures are completed and strained, you can take them singly or combined. "Kind of like the old pharmacist," says Kirsten. You can use mature tinctures to make any combination you feel you need for healing. It would be prudent to do some research into what you are combining and why. However, once tinctures have been combined, you are now limited because you cannot use them individually or in other combinations. For this reason, it is a good idea to only combine small amounts, as needed. Tinctures should only be combined when they are mature.

QUESTION: Can I combine tinctures made with different menstruums?

ANSWER: Yes. *Menstruum* is the word herbalists use to describe the liquid used to create an herbal tincture—alcohol, glycerin, or vinegar. Tinctures made with different menstruums can be combined. However, these should be used in a short period of time because, while alcohol tinctures have a shelf life of years, glycerin has a shelf life of two years and vinegar one year.

QUESTION: Can I combine dried herbs to create a tincture?

ANSWER: Yes, you can combine dried herbs into a specific formula when creating a tincture. For example, when making her tincture for lower bowel health (see Remedies chapter), Kirsten mixes the dried herbs first, making sure the menstruum ratio is correct for the ounces of dried herbs she uses. "There is no harm in that," she says. "It just limits my ability to use each herb individually for other things."

NOTES

1. Pedanius Dioscorides, *Book Five: Of Vines and Wines*, trans. Tess Anne Osbaldeston, accessed March 24, 2014, http://www.ibidispress.scriptmania.com/index.html.

2. Debra St Clair, *The Herbal Medicine Cabinet* (Berkeley: Celestial Arts, 1997).

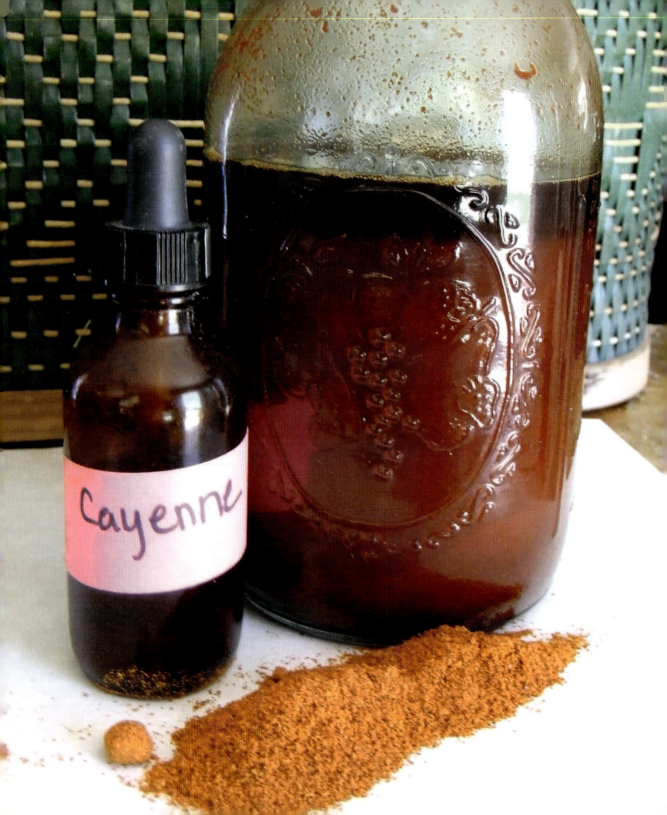

CHAPTER 8
CAYENNE
SCIENTIFIC NAMES
Capsicum annuum **OR** *Capsicum frutescens*

There are three herbs that Kirstin considers to be the most important herbs you need to have in your closet. These include cayenne, lobelia, and comfrey.

Cayenne is a hot red garden pepper. It is grown in the backyard garden and is usually green when mature and red when dried. To create your own cayenne powder, clean the peppers (wearing gloves) and scrape out the seeds and pith. Dry completely in a 200-degree oven, and then crush or blend into a powder. Cayenne peppers come in many shapes, colors, sizes, and heat levels, but few cayenne pepper varieties are the true medicinal variety. For true, guaranteed pure, non-hybrid, non-GMO medicinal cayenne seeds, see SeedRenaissance.com.

Cayenne does everything. It evens out your blood pressure. When you think about blood, you should think about cayenne. I use it often. I take it almost every day. The number one food for blood is cayenne—if you are bleeding, if your nose is bleeding, if you are having a heart attack, if your face is red, if your blood pressure is changing, you can use cayenne. If you have a bloody nose and stuff cayenne up your nose, the sensation is intense, but the herb helps. Cayenne can even be used to help prevent shock.

The Complete Herbal, published in 1653 by physician and botanist Nicholas Culpeper, says this about cayenne (which he called guinea pepper): ". . . they burn and inflame the mouth and throat so extremely that it is hard to be endured, and if it be outwardly applied to the skin in any part of the body, it will exulcerate and raise it as if it had been burnt with fire, or scalded with hot water… if any shall with their hands touch their face or eyes, it will cause so great an inflammation that it will not be remedied in a long time… given as one of the highest stimulants in cold sluggish phlegmatic disorders."

WARNINGS

Cayenne can burn the eyes and irritate the skin. Handle with care. Cayenne can cause a burning sensation in open wounds and sores and can be difficult to wash off. Do not apply to open wounds or sores. Cayenne does not dissolve easily, so use vinegar to get it off skin.

Cayenne is used to treat bloody noses, heart attacks, shock, nerves, and ear infection.

Kirsten says "Never go lower than 35,000 Scoville units for medicinal cayenne. Ninety [thousand] is high. Cayenne is something you need to get used to taking. Your body will get used to it and build up to it. Also, you can't always believe the Scoville units labels on cayenne if you purchase it. Sometimes a cayenne labeled 90,000 Scoville is not hot and sometimes a 35,000 is hotter. Normally, the hotter the cayenne, the more medicinal it is."

Cayenne can be used to stop nosebleeds or bleeding in any form. For nosebleeds, snort a pinch of cayenne into the bleeding nostril.

Cayenne has the ability to equal out blood pressure. It can be taken in tincture form or powder form for this use.

"Steve used it recently when he sliced his finger on a razor blade and was bleeding profusely," says Kirsten of her husband. "He took a dropper full of cayenne and the bleeding stopped. It was very hot and uncomfortable but it worked!" Cayenne may be useful in an emergency to temporarily treat a heart attack, if no other medical help is available.

"One of my teachers was learning about cayenne and there was an accident in front of his house," says Kirsten. "He immediately helped the person stop their internal bleeding by administering cayenne tincture before any help could arrive. He was told he had helped save the man's life."

Cayenne tincture is widely used to bring heat to the body for treating colds, flu, and pain. It can be taken internally and externally for these uses. Cayenne is also used as a daily tonic to encourage general health with apple cider vinegar in a glass of water. Cayenne can be made into a salve, using the salve recipe in this book, which is very warming and excellent for bruises as well as aches and pains.

When we have an injury, it is usually recommended to ice it. Heat is beneficial as well. Generally, you will want to rotate heat with ice. This allows the swelling to decrease while allowing healing to continue. A person usually knows when to trade out the ice for the cayenne salve, but five minutes of each is a good place to start.

Dose: If you have never taken cayenne before, start with one drop of cayenne tincture in Shock Tea (recipe below).

HOW TO TAKE CAYENNE

Take as a straight tincture, or mixed with other herbal tinctures, or diluted with water or herbal tea with honey. Do not take cayenne in a capsule because it can burn or damage the stomach.

Shock tea

This recipe is meant to prevent a person from going into shock. If a person is already in shock, they should not be given anything to drink, including shock tea. Call for medical help.

- 1 teaspoon cayenne powder (or, if you are new to cayenne, use only a trace of powder or 1–2 drops cayenne tincture)

- 1 tablespoon honey

- 1 tablespoon apple cider vinegar

- 1 cup water

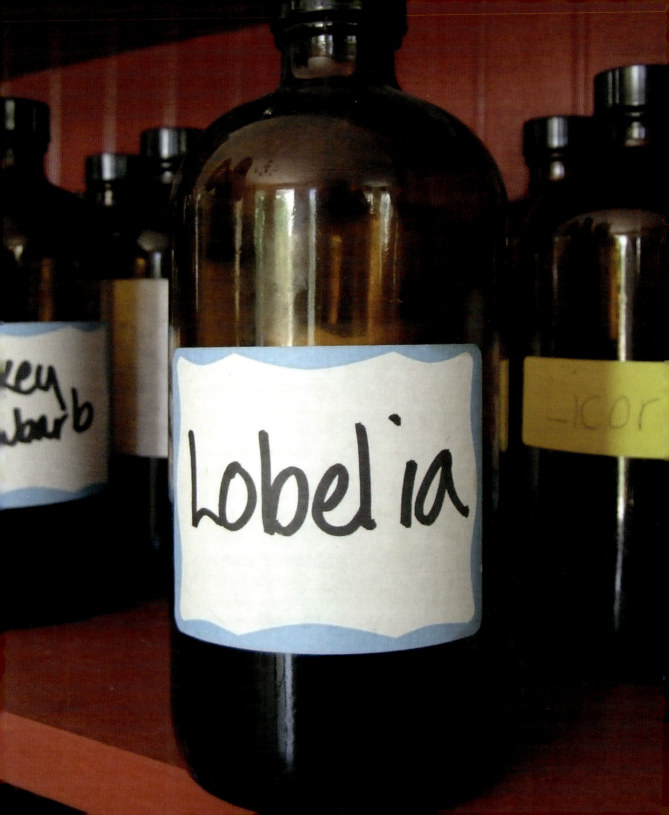

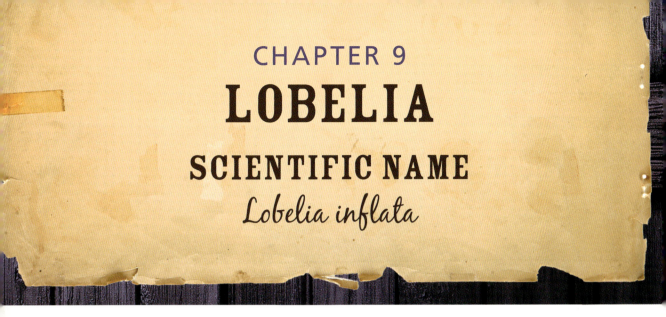

CHAPTER 9
LOBELIA
SCIENTIFIC NAME
Lobelia inflata

Lobelia is among the most powerful of all medicinal herbs and should be used respectfully. Lobelia has been called "The Thinking Herb" because of its aptitude for boosting the power of other herbs and helping them better perform their healing work. You can add lobelia to many herbal remedies to boost the effectiveness of those remedies. Lobelia is not used by itself. It usually accompanies another herb. You can add 3 to 10 drops of lobelia tincture to any medicinal herbal tea.

Part of the plant used: Leaves and seeds. (The best time to use the plant is after the leaves begin to turn yellow. This is when there is the most oil in the seed and plant).

Plant description:

There are many different varieties of lobelia sold for gardening and flower beds, with flowers ranging from blue to red to white. But there is only one medicinal species of lobelia, and that is *Lobelia inflata*, which is also called Lobelia Official. *Official* is the historic scientific name used to designate herbs used medicinally. Because there are more than 400 varieties of lobelia that are not medicinal, be sure when planting and growing lobelia for medicinal purposes that you have a guaranteed medicinal variety, such as is sold by SeedRenaissance.com.

HOW TO PREPARE LOBELIA

Tea

Fresh or dried lobelia can be used on its own or with other fresh or dried herbs to make a medicinal tea. You can regularly add a pinch of lobelia to any medicinal tea you make.

Tincture

Dried lobelia may be made into a tincture using vinegar, using the recipe in the Tinctures chapter of this book. Apple cider vinegar has a special relationship with lobelia, meaning lobelia seems to work better medicinally when combined with apple cider vinegar, for whatever reason. Once prepared, tincture of lobelia can be mixed with other mature tinctures for medicinal use.

Salad

A pinch of fresh lobelia leaves may be added to any regular lunch or dinner salad as a method of getting this herb into the body to do its work.

HOW TO USE LOBELIA

What makes lobelia so important is its amazing emetic properties and its ability to relax and clear mucus from the body. Those are three of the top priorities in the healing process.

Fluid extracts of lobelia are usually stronger. Lobelia can be used in two ways. One, as a stimulant, to help the body move and expel toxins. And two, as a relaxant.

Lobelia in large doses can be used to induce vomiting as needed.

If you take too much lobelia tincture, you will be throwing up for a long time. When used to make someone vomit, it is accompanied by peppermint to make the stomach feel better by the retching action. It is very quick and powerful. When someone is vomiting or expectorating out of control, like my mom was with cancer, a few drops of lobelia tincture stopped that action so she could rest. But stopping the vomit is not always recommended, because vomiting usually has a purpose.

As a general rule, lobelia should always be preceded by or given in combination with another stimulant to help the body move out toxins. Peppermint or cayenne proceed lobelia when it is being used as a stimulant. This means taking a tea or tincture of peppermint or cayenne about 15 minutes before taking tea or tincture of lobelia if you are using it as a stimulant. The peppermint tea is soothing to the stomach and is also a more stable stimulant. When used as a relaxant, do not combine with cayenne or goldenseal, but with a more diffusive agent, such as ginger.

- In small doses it can be used to stop vomiting.

- Lobelia tincture is added to other tinctures to help cut mucus in the body as an expectorant.

- Lobelia is best stored as a tincture, and not as a dried herb, due to the volatile oils in both the herb and the seed.

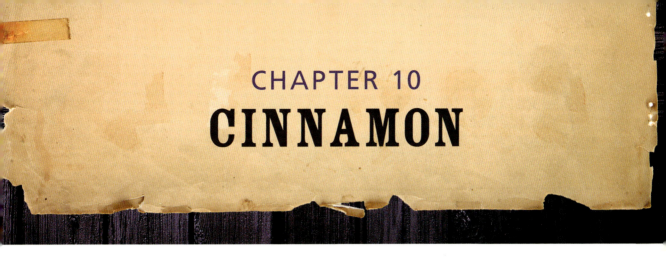

CHAPTER 10
CINNAMON

Common cinnamon, the kind found in every grocery store, has health benefits in the same category as cayenne and ginger, but tastes better. Volumes of research exist on the medicinal benefits of cinnamon. It has been used by the Chinese and the Egyptians for many years. It is even mentioned in the Bible, as food and medicine. At one time, cinnamon was reportedly worth more than gold. It was among the first traded goods between Europe and Asia.

TYPES OF CINNAMON

Cassia Cinnamon

Most cinnamon found in your local grocery is cassia cinnamon. If you are going to use cinnamon as a medicine, without risk to the liver, you will need to be aware of what kind you are buying. cassia cinnamon is not recommended. There have been many tests in Europe that suggest cassia cinnamon may contain a dose of the molecule coumarin, which can be detrimental to the liver. Extensive studies have suggested that cassia cinnamon may be beneficial to those with diabetes, as well as having many of the same benefits of Ceylon cinnamon. However the risk of coumarin overdose outweighs the benefits.

Cinnamomum zylanicum (Ceylon Cinnamon)

"I would suggest the use of Ceylon cinnamon," says Kirsten. "Ceylon cinnamon is antioxidant, anti-microbial, a blood sugar stabilizer, anthelmintic when used with wormwood and black walnut or cloves, and has been used for centuries to help alleviate digestive disorders. It is used as a warming tonic, alongside ginger, clover, peppercorn, astragalus, and licorice. It has also been used as a free radical scavenger and to lower blood pressure.

"Many people have found benefits by having a cup of warm water with honey and cinnamon before bed and in the morning as a way of lowering their insulin levels and managing their weight. I have only used this for a short time; however, I have seen the benefits, or maybe I just enjoy the tea. One teaspoon of cinnamon per day is recommended for medicinal benefits."

Studies on Ceylon cinnamon suggest numerous beneficial health effects of this spice, including anti-inflammatory properties, anti-microbial activity, reducing cardiovascular disease, boosting cognitive function, and reducing risk of colonic cancer, as well as anti-parasitic, antioxidant, and free radical scavenging properties. Ceylon cinnamon may also inhibit some of the physical hallmarks of Alzheimer's disease, lower blood glucose, lower cholestrol, and lower blood pressure, according to a survey of medicinal cinnamon research at Biomedcentral.com.

For more information about the medicinal benefits of cinnamon, go to Biomedcentral.com and type "true cinnamon" into the search bar to access a survey of cinnamon research titled "Medicinal properties of 'true' cinnamon (*Cinnamomum zeylanicum*): a systematic review."[1]

NOTES

1. Priyanga Ranasinghe et al., "Medicinal Properties of 'True' Cinnamon (*Cinnamomum zeylanicum*): a Systematic Review," October 22, 2013, doi: 10.1186/1472-6882-13-275.

One teaspoon of Ceylon cinnamon per day is recommended for medicinal benefits.

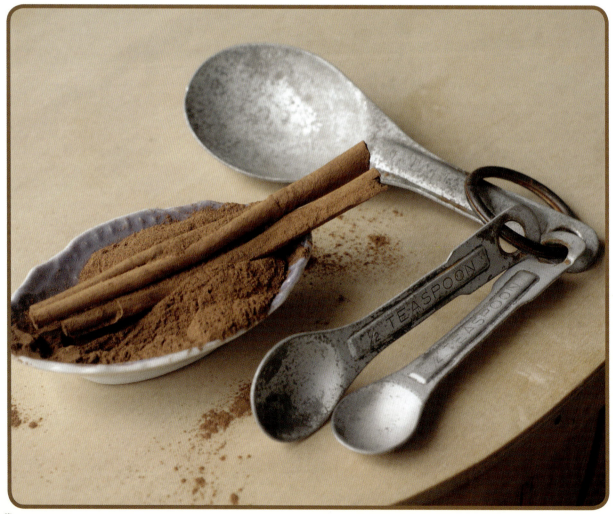

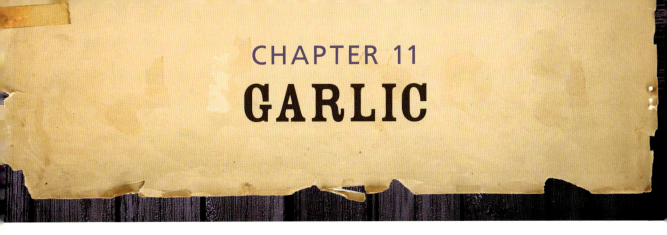

CHAPTER 11
GARLIC

arlic has been used for thousands of years as an antibiotic. It kills viruses, bacteria, parasites, and even fungi. There has been research done on garlic and how it benefits heart health. Studies show garlic helps fight some cancers from growing. Adding fresh garlic to any dish is beneficial. One clove per day can be used as a preventative to many illnesses.

ALLICIN: WAITING FOR SCIENCE TO CATCH UP TO HERBAL MEDICINE

The more the world learns about the scientific evidence for the medicinal powers of garlic and onions, the more fascinating the studies become. Both vegetables have the ability to produce a powerful compound called *allicin*. Equally fascinating is how much herbalists knew about this medicine—before scientists had a name for it, or any understanding of how it works.

Allicin is a trickster. It is only formed when garlic, onions, leeks, and chives are crushed, cut, or chewed. This triggers an enzyme called *alliinase*, which causes allicin to form. Although allicin has been studied extensively, exactly how it works is still unknown—but however it works, science has shown repeatedly that allicin has significant disease-fighting gumption.

Tests have shown that the enzyme that allows allicin to form is destroyed by heat, according to Oregon State University research. Also, the half-life of allicin in crushed garlic at 73 degrees Fahrenheit is two and a half days. Allicin breaks down into two other medicinal compounds, called *ajoene* and *vinyl-dithiins*—but only when the garlic is mixed with oil as it breaks down. Despite testing, ajoene and vinyl-dithiins have never been detected in human blood, urine, or stool, which seems to mean they are metabolized by the body very fast. In plain language, this appears to mean our bodies really likes these two medicines. Evidence shows that these compounds have big medicinal skills, including inhibiting bad cholesterol, heart disease, inflammation, and certain cancers. These compounds are anti-viral, anti-fungal, anti-inflammatory and antioxidant, according to Oregon State University, which has compiled an impressive array of research into allicin. You can access this research by going to lpi.oregonstate.edu and clicking "Micronutrient Information Center," then clicking "Foods/Beverages," and then choosing "Garlic."[1]

All of this is important medicine that is available right at our fingertips. Keep in mind that everything mentioned above is just the benefits of garlic oil—not including fresh garlic, extracted garlic, or garlic tincture, which all have their own long list of associated

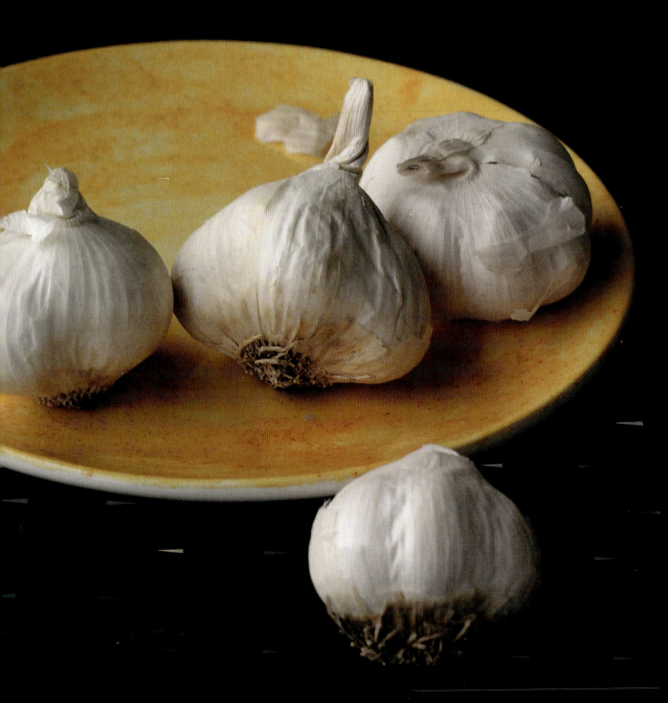

compounds and health benefits. All of the science behind allicin and the other organosulfur compounds associated with garlic, onions, leeks, and chives could easily fill a book.

To us, this science is useful because it confirms what herbalists have long known—that garlic is powerful medicine.

Imagine if the world had refused to use garlic until science could explain its virtues?

The science of garlic as a curative is just another reminder that it is not always wise to wait until science can explain the details of natural healing. We would still be waiting—and we'd be sick. There is no doubt about the relative benefit of costly and extensive medicinal studies, but garlic alone should put to rest any doubt that natural medicine is simply folklore or wishful thinking. We need to take better advantage of, and have more faith in, the "scientific testing" our ancestors conducted on themselves for centuries, showing the clear and present competence of natural healing. We are not always benefited by waiting for some company to tell us what is, and is not, medicine.

MEDICINAL GARLIC

Anytime Kirsten's family is suffering from illness, she brings out the garlic. She adds it to food, rubs it on the body, or takes it with honey and cayenne.

"Garlic has never failed us," says Kirsten. Nor has it failed the thousands who have depended on this herb for the past 5,000 years.

How to Make Garlic Oil

- 1–2 heads of garlic, peeled
- Olive oil

STEP 1. Put the garlic cloves in a half-pint glass jar. Pour enough olive oil to barely cover them.

STEP 2. Pour garlic and oil into the blender and blend. Pour back into the jar.

STEP 3. Cover the jar with cheesecloth, secured with a rubber band or canning jar ring. It is essential that you do NOT cover the jar with a regular lid, because botulism will set in. Botulism is a toxin produced by several strains of bacteria that thrive in food stored in a high-moisture, low-salt, low-acid environment without oxygen or refrigeration.[2]

Garlic oil covered with cheesecloth allows oxygen to prevent the growth of botulism.

Your mixture should sit for a week without shaking or stirring. You can then strain out the garlic pulp and use the oil medicinally.

One of the best ways to add garlic to your daily diet is to use Kirsten's salad dressing recipe.

Kirsten's Medicinal Garlic Salad Dressing

- 2 cloves garlic
- ½ onion
- 2 cups oil
- ¾ cup vinegar
- Salt, pepper, and spices of your choice.

In a blender, combine the ingredients until smooth. Serve over salad. When adding spices or herbs to this salad dressing, Kirsten recommends "pot herbs," which are a combination of your favorite herbs all jumbled together. This is a great way to individualize your dressing. Kirsten often starts with basil and marjoram.

Garlic Strep Throat Remedy

- 3 cloves garlic, peeled
- 2 tablespoons honey
- 1 teaspoon (or as much as you can handle) cayenne pepper powder.

Mash garlic into honey and stir in cayenne. Take one-quarter teaspoon or one-half teaspoon every hour. Let the thick mix sit on the throat for 45 minutes, and then drink water (never milk) or other healthful liquid for 15 minutes. Repeat for 24 hours. It is best not to bother an ill person while they are sleeping, but they should use this remedy as often as possible in order to kill the strep.

Garlic for Respiratory Illness

If someone in your home is ill with a respiratory sickness, have the person take a hot bath and drink plenty of hot liquid, preferably Feverfew tea or Red Raspberry tea, at least a quart, preferably several. When they cannot handle the hot bath any longer, wrap them in a cold sheet and put them to bed. Rub garlic oil on their feet and then place socks on their feet. Let them sweat this out overnight. In the morning, the sick person should shower, and then rinse their body with apple cider vinegar as a cleanser.

This treatment is called the Cold Sheet Treatment. It is based on the ancient treatment of hydrotherapy. Dr. John Raymond Christopher, the renowned herbalist, gave the name to this treatment that has been practiced by many, including Kirsten, with extremely high rate of success. The use of diaphoretics (herbs that make you sweat) such as red raspberry leaf,

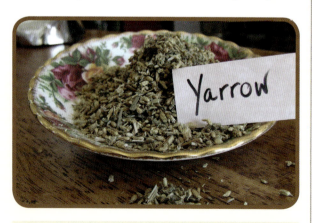

The use of diaphoretics (herbs that make you sweat) such as red raspberry leaf, boneset, yarrow, or chamomile is essential to the Cold Sheet Treatment.

boneset, yarrow, or chamomile, drunk by the quart, is essential to this treatment.

It is helpful to remember that when someone has a fever, temperature is not the enemy. Fevers have a purpose. Temperatures increase the action of the macrophage, which fight illness. However, a fever that is dry, meaning there is too little liquid in the body, can be very dangerous.

Garlic Oil Chest Rub for Respiratory Illness

To help ease the symptoms of infection in the chest, rub into the chest of the sick person a dropper-full of garlic oil. This is safe and effective for both children and adults.

Garlic Oil for Ear Infections

To treat ear infections, put a couple of drops of garlic oil in the affected ear. The sick person should tilt their head to help keep the oil drops in the ear canal. Put new drops in every couple of hours, as needed, until the infection goes away. You may need to place some cotton in the ear so the garlic oil does not drain out.

Another way to attack ear infections with garlic is to mix garlic oil, mullein tincture for pain, and lobelia tincture. Put this mixture both on the outside of the ear and inside the ear, then close the ear with a cotton ball.

Another option: Use garlic oil mixed with astragalus oil for ear infections. This works because astragalus supports the immune system

Garlic to Fight Yeast Infection

As medicine for a yeast infection, take a clove of garlic wrapped in gauze and insert it into the vagina, with a part of the gauze within reach. This can cure a

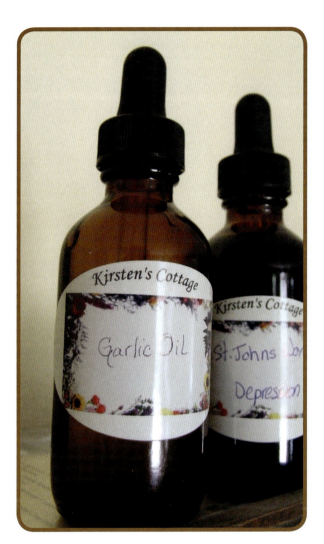

yeast infection in a very short period of time. Wrapping a garlic clove in gauze is called a bolus. A garlic bolus can be changed once or twice a day. Use the bolus treatment for several days, or until there are no symptoms of the yeast infection. You may ask, why would garlic, an antibiotic, cure yeast, which is often caused by antibiotics? It is anti-fungal, anti-inflammatory, and an antioxidant. These are all good reasons why garlic works.

Garlic to Fight Acne

Kirsten has successfully used slightly bruised garlic directly on acne with pleasing results. Rub the bruised garlic directly on the affected skin. This works because of garlic's anti-bacterial properties and the allicin that it contains

NOTES

1. "Garlic and Organosulfur Compounds" Linus Pauling Institute, accessed October 21, 2014, http://lpi.oregonstate.edu/infocenter/phytochemicals/garlic/.
2. P. Kendall, "Botulism," May 2012, accessed October 21, 2014, http://www.ext.colostate.edu/pubs/foodnut/09305.html.

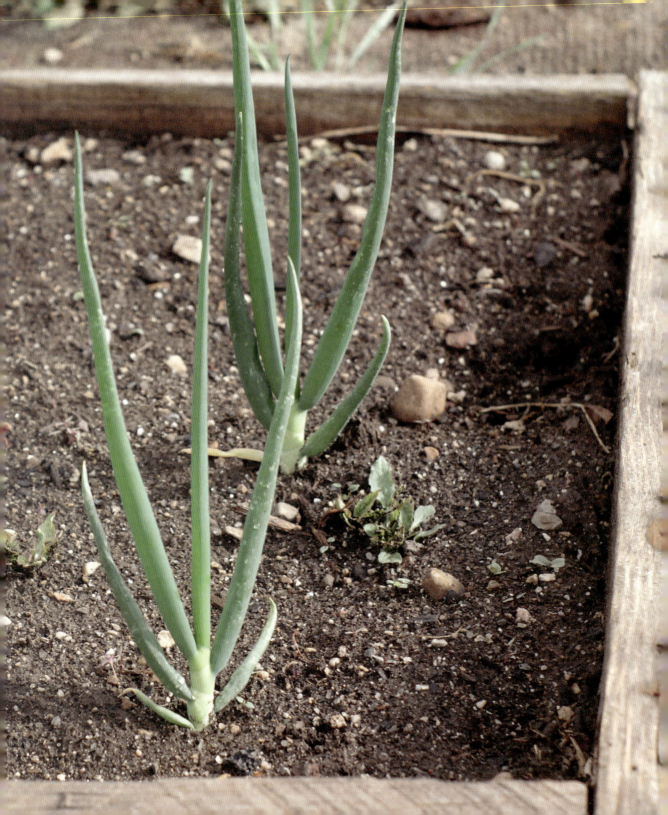

CHAPTER 12
THE COMMON ONION

No herbal book would be complete without mentioning the household onion. The common garden onion has enormous medicinal benefits and should be more widely used as preventative medicine and also as a healing aid.

THE DRAWING ONION

There are a group of herbs that have the power of drawing, which means they can draw out or neutralize the venom of bees and wasps, and even help the body eject splinters. The onion has a wonderful drawing power and can be used on children and adults to help immediately calm and sooth the pain of a sting or bug bite.

"When I was a very young girl, I was playing down at a neighbor's house, and I was stung by a bee on the foot," says Kirsten. "I was frantic. My neighbor's mother came out of the house and brought half an onion with her. Taking my foot, she placed the onion on it and held it there. I thought this woman was crazy but was too intimidated to tell her so. Within moments, my food no longer stung and I was able to go play. I never forgot that onion, nor her kindness."

Onion as Mucus Fighter

Garden onions have a robust ability to help clear mucus out of the respiratory system just by laying them on top of the chest. Begin by cutting an onion and heating it until it becomes soft or slippery. Wrap the onion in gauze if you have some, as this will help the onion stay in place. Apply olive oil to the chest and then add the onion poultice on top. Wrap an ace bandage around the chest to keep it from moving, or with a small child, a tight t-shirt will work. Change out the onions after they have lost their heat. This can be done throughout the day and night until there is noticeable relief. This method can help anyone—child or adult—who is struggling to get proper air. Simply putting a sliced onion on a plate near your bed when you are sick can also help adults and children breath easier.

At Caleb's house, whenever there is someone with congestion, a runny nose, a cough, sinus pressure, or a sore throat, priority number one is to cook with onions—in stew, in omelets, in soup, in onion rings—whatever it takes to get onions into the body. Onions are a simple but forceful power for cutting mucus in the body. Eat them. Put the on the chest. Put them near the bed—do all of these things. Put onions to the test for your family.

"So many of our illnesses stem from the overproduction of mucus," says Kirsten. "If we can eliminate the mucus, we eliminate the illness. There is a reason people often suggest not to drink milk or eat milk product when ill, because encourages the body to produce mucus. It might be wise for us to determine what items in our lives are producing mucus in the first place and then eliminate, or at least be careful with, those foods, before we become ill."

Onions for Sinus Pain

Caleb has a lifetime of experience with sinusitis. His sinus congestion leads to migraines so powerful

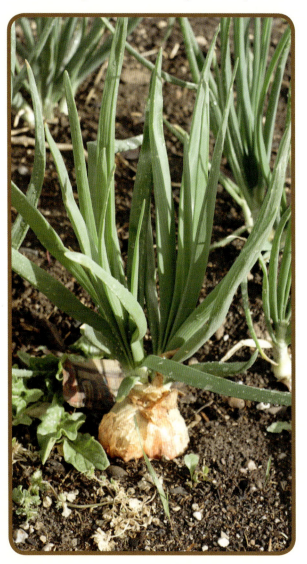

they have left him unconscious on the floor—you can read more about this is the chapter of this book called "The Forgotten Art of Quarantine." Caleb has learned through hard experience that if you are a person prone to sinus infections, prevention is salvation. Caleb's case is so acute that he cannot blow his nose if he has any congestion at all—blowing his nose creates vacuums in his sinus with sharp, instant pain that only grows—and only ends in an immobilizing migraine. Instead of blowing his nose, he has learned from hard experience that he has to let his nose run—this is the only chance of clearing the congestion safely.

Here's where onions come in. Onions help cut mucus from the sinus. The same power that can make you cry when you cut an onion can also make your sinus "cry" too—and what a joyful relief it is. In the worst cases, putting a towel over your head so you can inhale the odor of onion is helpful.

For the worst cases, heat a chopped or sliced onion in a cup of water on the stove until it is steaming and then put it under the towel to breathe in relief—just keep your eyes closed or you will be crying too.

"Simply chopping up a few raw onions may be enough to clear your sinuses," according to LiveStrong.com. "Since heat and steam are other home remedies for congestion, you may want to add chunks of raw onion to hot broth. Sip the broth in a cup to bring the steam and onion close to your nose. You don't have to actually eat raw onion to benefit from its antihistamine and anti-inflammatory properties."[1]

In cold and flu season, you can set chopped onions near your bed at night to help ease congested breathing. However, do not put onions near small children at night, because the vapors of the onion might sting or affect their eyes, and they won't be able to tell you.

QUERCETIN

The naturally occurring medicine found in onions is a molecule called quercetin. "Quercetin acts like an antihistamine and an anti-inflammatory, and may help protect against heart disease and cancer," according to the University of Maryland Medical Center's "Complementary and Alternative Medicine Guide." "Quercetin can also help stabilize the cells that release histamine in the body and thereby have an anti-inflammatory effect."[2]

Quercetin occurs naturally in red wine, grapefruit, onions, apples, and black tea, and in smaller amounts in leafy green vegetables and beans. "Quercetin has an antioxidant and anti-inflammatory activity" and "inhibits the growth of certain malignant (cancer) cells in vitro . . . and also displays unique anticancer properties. Quercetin is a natural compound that blocks substances involved in

allergies . . . Quercetin is a safe, natural therapy that may be used as primary therapy or in conjunction with conventional methods," according to a research published in 2006 by the Boston University School of Medicine.[3]

NOTES

1. Carolyn Robbins, "Does a Cut-up Onion Clear Sinus?," December 18, 2013, accessed October 21, 2014, http://www.livestrong.com/article/535180-does-a-cut-up-onion-clear-sinuses/.

2. "Quercetin," University of Maryland Medical Center, accessed October 21, 2014, http://umm.edu/health/medical/altmed/supplement/quercetin#ixzz2xli9IMc2.

3. Y. B. Shaik et al., "Role of Quercetin (a Natural Herbal Compound) in Allergy and Inflammation," *Journal of Biological Regulators and Homeostatic Agents* 20, no. 3–4 (2006): 47–52, http://www.ncbi.nlm.nih.gov/pubmed/18187018%20.

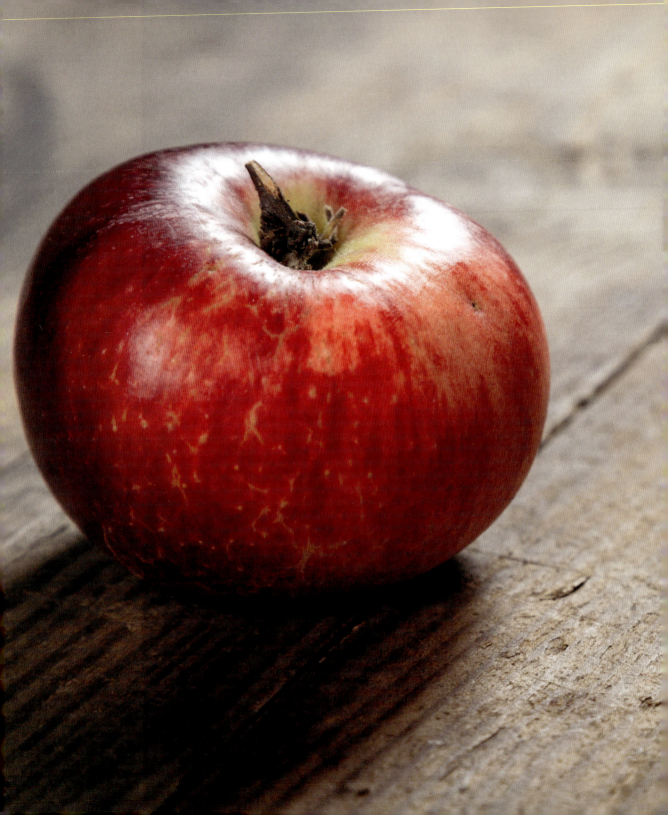

CHAPTER 13
APPLE CIDER VINEGAR

I take apple cider vinegar every single day," says Kirsten. "Apple cider vinegar is a balm to the circulatory tract. I am talking medicinal apple cider vinegar. I would suggest making your own or using Bragg's. Their vinegar is living vinegar. It is undistilled, organic, and raw. It still has part of the "mother" in the vinegar they sell."

Apple cider vinegar helps to clean the arteries of the calcium deposits that are layered there.

"It has been used for the past 3,000 years, since the Egyptians, and anyone with any sense continues the practice," says Kirsten. "It was brought across the sea to prevent scurvy and carried into many wars. It is difficult to get down raw, but worth all the funny faces you will make doing so! Try it in every salad you eat or pour onto any food. I like to drink mine in a glass of water with honey and a touch of cayenne. That way I am getting the benefits of an antibiotic and heat to cleanse my capillaries and my heart, while helping to maintain the acid-alkaline balance in my body. There is a reason soldiers have used it to stay strong. Go apple cider vinegar!"

Apple cider vinegar has a one-year shelf life.

Kirsten's mother, Marilyn Gilbert, has become an expert in making her own vinegar. Here is her recipe:

TO MAKE VINEGAR FROM SCRATCH

"Easy Method"

STEP 1. Start with a glass or stainless steel container. If you use a metal container, use only stainless steel. A container with a wide mouth is best. The vinegar culture can be made from anything containing starch or sugar. Any food that has sugar as part of its makeup is the best—think of fresh fruit, beets and similar such foods but in juice form, either fresh or frozen juice (not canned). You will want the juice—not the whole fruit or vegetable. To keep the liquid from evaporating too quickly, Marilyn suggests covering the container with cheesecloth.

STEP 2. Obtain a "vinegar culture," either at a home brew store or at a grocery store that sells unpasteurized, unfiltered vinegar. You will also need a dark, warm place to keep the container. One place to keep a container warm and dark is at the top of a covered shelf in the kitchen; I have seen one maker put the container on the top of the water heater! The major word is warm, not hot.

STEP 3. Pour about one quart of the starter into the container. Add about the same amount of the juice. Do not cover the container completely. Put the container in the warm, dark place and check it every two to three weeks. Once it reaches the strength you like, you can strain it if necessary and bottle it in small bottles. Do not use this for a period of approximately six months. Once you have made your own vinegar, you will probably never buy the commercial bottled vinegar again!

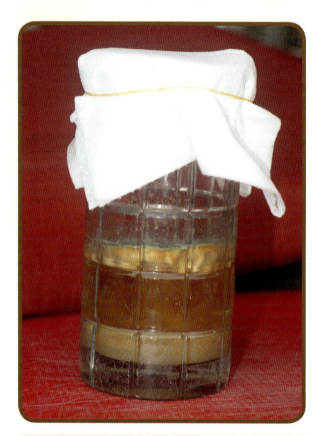

Caleb Warnock's homemade mother-of-vinegar using winter apples from the root cellar.

TO MAKE VINEGAR FROM SCRATCH

"Longer Method"

This method begins by creating a "mother of vinegar" culture from scratch.

STEP 1. Place 2 tablespoons of unfiltered, unpasteurized vinegar into a bowl and add half a bottle of wine or cider. Place this in a warm sunny place (not a dark place) for two weeks. This will form a skin that creates the necessary bacteria. This "mother" can now turn wine or any other alcohol into vinegar. After the mother has formed, skim it off and place it in another wide-mouthed container. Follow the directions given in the "easy method," but after

one month, strain the liquid and remove the mother. The mother can be kept and used again indefinitely as long as some kind of alcohol is added to it.

QUESTIONS AND ANSWERS ABOUT MAKING HOMEMADE VINEGAR

QUESTION: **How long will the mother of vinegar last?**

ANSWER: The mother will last a long time if you periodically feed it with the same kind of alcohol you initially started it with—red wine, white wine, hard cider. After your vinegar has matured for at least three months, add wine at about one-fourth the volume of the main culture, with a small amount of water, every one to two months. The culture should always be kept in a dark, warm spot.

QUESTION: **Can I make homemade vinegar using just apples?**

ANSWER: Yes. Published in 1961, *The Natural Foods Cookbook* by Beatrice Trum Hunter suggests simply washing and then cutting up whole tart apples (stems and all).[1] Mush the chunks, or pulp them through a potato ricer, and then strain the juice through muslin cloth into a clean glass jar. Cover the jar with a triple thickness of cheesecloth (secured with string or a rubber band) and put it in a dark, warm place for six months. Strain the vinegar and use. You can keep the mother on top to start a new vinegar. The new vinegar will form faster because you already have a mother of vinegar.

NOTES

1. Beatrice Trum Hunter, *The Natural Foods Cookbook* (New York: Touchstone, 1969).

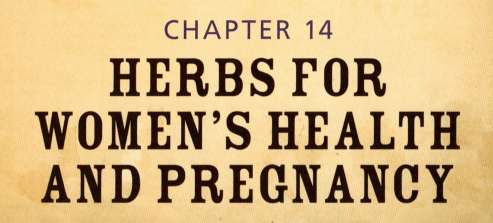

CHAPTER 14
HERBS FOR WOMEN'S HEALTH AND PREGNANCY

RED RASPBERRY LEAF

Rubus idaeus

Red Raspberry Leaf is exactly what is sounds like—the leaves of the popular berry bush that so many gardeners have in their backyards, producing a bounty of red summer berries. But did you know the leaves of this plant are useful medicine? Red raspberry leaf is a simple herb, but has helped many people in pregnancy and sickness and is known as "the woman's herb."

Menses Pain

To manage and dull menses pain, use Red raspberry leaf tea on its own, or combine it with cramp bark tea to target the uterine muscles and help them relax.

Mucus Fighter

Red raspberry leaf helps remove mucus from the body, so it is very good to drink when taking a hot bath. It is often used to bring the body into balance

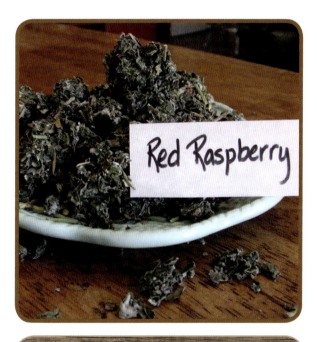

Red Raspberry

Parts used medicinally

Leaves. Harvesting too many leaves can damage the plant and affect the berry harvest. Pick no more than every third leaf on a plant.

when our internal systems are off-kilter because they are under attack from viruses or bacteria. Red raspberry leaf can help the body restore balance by inducing sweat to clean itself out. As you read in the Garlic chapter of this book, red raspberry leaf tea is an important part of the Cold Sheet Treatment. In that instance, the tea is used for both men, women, and children.

Recipe for Red Raspberry Leaf Tea

"This is a tea that can be drunk by the gallon," says Kirsten. "When I am sick, I drink only red raspberry tea, and forgo any solid food as long as I can to clear the mucus, and thus the illness, from my body. It is mild enough for any age. I cannot think of any illness that would not benefit from red raspberry tea. Try mixing two-thirds raspberry tea and one-third peppermint tea for a wonderful summer treat. I usually add a little honey or stevia as well. This is a perfect example of making herbs part of our daily diet. This is about prevention."

- ¼ cup dried leaves OR ⅓ cup fresh leaves
- 1 quart water

OPTION 1. Put water in a pot on the stove top. Stir in herbs. As soon as the water begins to boil around the edges, turn off the heat. Let sit for five minutes. Strain and drink as wanted. You may add a pinch of stevia for sweetening as desired.

OPTION 2. Bring water to a boil and turn off heat. Pour the water over the herbs and let steep for five minutes. Strain and drink as wanted. You may add a pinch of stevia for sweetening as desired.

CRAMPS

Tea made of cramp bark, mixed with a couple of drops of lobelia tea, is used to treat cramps. If the cramps are severe, you can add a few more drops of lobelia tincture, but it is very powerful, so don't add more than five or six drops.

HERBS FOR HORMONES

"If you are not taking red raspberry leaf, change your life and start taking red raspberry!" says Kirsten. "If you are a woman from 10 to 60 years old, your hormones are up and down. There is nothing wrong with drinking a half-gallon of red raspberry tea a day."

Anyone who is struggling with hormone imbalance as a teen or during pregnancy, during menses, or during menopause can benefit from red raspberry leaf.

"It is used to regulate hormones from the beginning of menses through the end," says Kirsten. "You will find this especially helpful in the teen years, or pregnancy and menopause, when hormones are changing."

Red raspberry leaf is also used for teen boys who are hormonal and can benefit from smoothing out their hormone balance.

There are also other herbal options for natural hormone relief:

- Tincture of wild yam leaf using any of the three tincture recipes in this book.
- Cream of wild yam leaf rubbed onto the body.

CALCIUM RECIPE

For anyone concerned about bone health or increasing their calcium intake, here is a recipe that will improve your calcium levels. Some people are not familiar with recipes that call for "parts" instead of specific measurements like cups or tablespoons. A recipe based on parts simply means that you can make a lot or a little, with the same recipe, as long as you are consistent in your ratios. For example, in the recipe below, "one part" might be a cup or a quart, and the fractional ingredients are adjusted according to how you define "one part".

- 1 part horsetail tincture
- 1 part oat straw tincture
- ⅛ part lobelia tincture

STEP 1. Mix tinctures and drink daily or as desired.

PREGNANCY

Red raspberry leaf can help calm the nausea that so often accompanies pregnancy, or even just common nausea from everyday illness.

"All herbs we discuss in this book are meant to be used in their natural form," says Kirsten. "I had a friend who asked me what I took for morning sickness. I explained the benefits of red raspberry tea and she decided to try it. She explained that it had not helped at all. I then saw the tea that she was taking. It was not the natural leaf tea of the red raspberry plant. It was a pre-packaged tea which included red dye. I do not recommend taking this kind of tea. When I saw what she was taking, I explained the difference in the teas. She began taking the regular red raspberry leaf tea in its natural form and her nausea was alleviated."

Extreme caution is necessary when taking any kind of herbs during pregnancy. Herbs can be powerful medicine, and many herbs should not be used during pregnancy.

Herbal Don'ts During Pregnancy

Peristalsis muscles are specialized muscles in our bodies that contract to move things along, for example, in the bowels and esophagus. Any herb that makes your peristalsis muscles move during pregnancy could start labor. These should not be used. These include pennyroyal and black cohosh.

Mother's Milk Flow

For nursing mothers trying to increase or extend their breast milk, use a tea of blessed thistle.

Stopping the Flow of Mother's Milk

"If you have lost a baby, one of the most painful things, not just emotionally, is that your milk has come in," says Kirsten. "Many women in that position have successfully used cabbage leaves. Just take out the middle of the cabbage and put the whole cabbage on your breasts and that will stop the milk. Or, put the raw cabbage leaves in your bra."

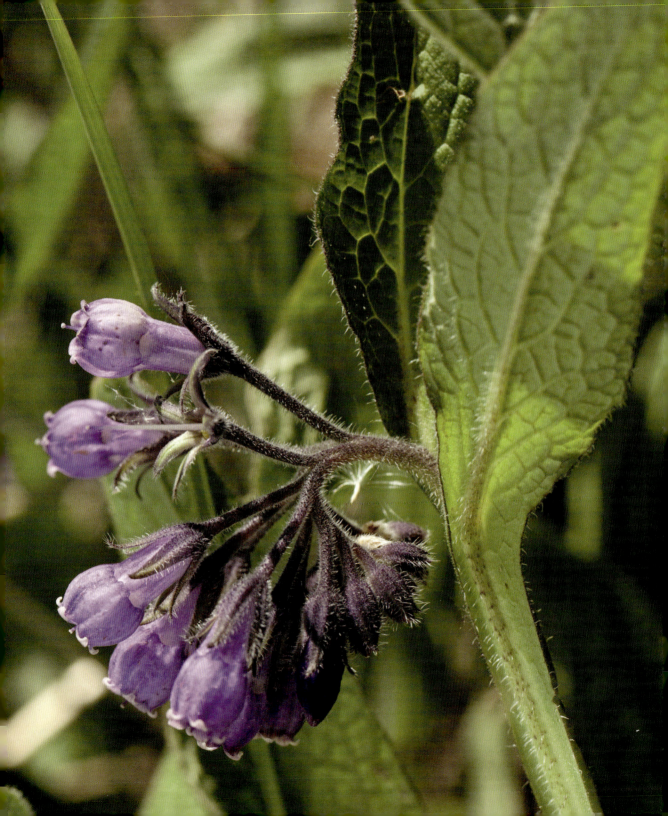

CHAPTER 15
HEALING FLESH AND BONES

COMFREY

Symphytum officinale

Kirsten's interest in medicinal comfrey prompted her to make it the subject of her thesis when she was working toward her master's certification from the School of Natural Healing, founded in 1953 by Dr. John R. Christopher.

"I love it," Kirsten says. "It is a cell proliferator, which means that it helps the body create cells. Everyone in the natural healing field has a comfrey story. It is also known as knitbone. It will knit the bones back together the way they are supposed to be. I always travel with comfrey. My kids absolutely love comfrey salve. They use it for everything."

Kirsten has her own comfrey story. She once went on a ropes course with her family. High in the

Parts used medicinally

The leaves, stalk, and root. The root is the most powerful. Do not use the young plant, which has paralyzing alkaloids. Use only the mature plant when it is two feet tall. If they are not that big, they are not ready for harvesting. Comfrey is also called *knitbone*.

air, she jumped off the pole holding her and, scared, grabbed the rope with her bare hand as she slide down to the ground.

"The rope went through my hand," Kirsten says. "I had comfrey with me and I put it on." Her hand healed fully and relatively quickly.

Though there are no ill effects with using comfrey externally, be cautious about using comfrey internally.

When taken as a tincture, comfrey can be particularly helpful against respiratory illness.

Comfrey Alkaloids

"The root and young leaves (of comfrey) contain a toxic alkaloid which, according to some modern research, may cause liver damage if taken in large amounts (more than the liver can process and eliminate). If the liver is congested or weak, it is better to use the mature leaf for internal use, avoiding the root and young leaf if possible. Generally, very large amounts are required to produce any harmful effect, so just be wise in your use of the root and young leaves," says Dr. John R. Christopher in his book *School of Natural Healing.*[1] Because of these studies, the FDA banned the sale of comfrey for internal use. They rarely cite the fact that the studies that support this finding took comfrey internally in very large amounts, more than any normal person would. That being said, the large leaves of the comfrey plant do not contain the toxic or paralyzing alkaloid. As with any herb, caution and wisdom must be your guide.

When deciding what part of the comfrey plant to use, know that the healing power of the plant is present in the old leaves, stronger in the whole plant, and greatest in the root.

Applying Comfrey to Wounds

When comfrey is applied to a wound, the wound will begin to heal, creating virgin white tissue.

When you see white, those are the new cells," says Kirsten. "Yellow cells are the infection. Do not take the comfrey off, and don't wash it off. Leave it on. It will become dust and the healing agent in the comfrey is absorbed into the skin."

New tissue begins to grow very quickly once comfrey salve has been applied to a wound, so wounds with infection require special caution.

"You need to be aware that if you have an open wound with infection, the comfrey will cover the

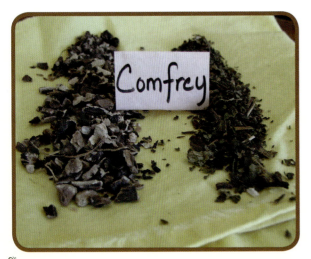

infection," trapping it in the body, says Kirsten. "So let the infection heal first. For most of the wounds you are going to come across in your lifetime, you don't need to worry about it."

Comfrey salve also helps minimize old scars. Simply apply the salve to the old scar daily until the scar fades.

Recipe for Comfrey Salve

- 2 oz. dried comfrey
- 8 oz. olive oil OR wheat germ oil
- ½ oz. beeswax (double this amount if you prefer a thicker salve)

OPTION 1. Heating pad method. Place comfrey and oil together in a covered cooking pot, making sure the herbs are stirred in and the oil is covering the herbs. Place the pot on a hot pad for 24 hours. The temperature should not exceed 110 degrees. Strain the oil. Add beeswax and stir until beeswax has melted and is incorporated into the mixture. Pour this into a container and let it harden. Keep a lid on the container when not in use.

OPTION 2. Crock pot method. If you have a crock pot with a "warm" setting (this is not the same as the "low" setting), then you can put the oil and herbs into a crock pot on this setting for 24 hours. Stir the oil and herbs together in the pot before turning on the heat, and make sure the oil is covering the herbs. Strain the oil. Add beeswax and stir until beeswax has melted and is incorporated into the mixture. Pour this into a container and let it harden. Keep a lid on the container when not in use.

OPTION 3. No-heat method. You can also make salve without heat by stirring comfrey and oil together and then putting the mix into a covered pot for two weeks. Strain the oil when it has the color and smell of the herb. Add melted beeswax and stir until beeswax is incorporated into the mixture. Pour this into a container and let it harden. Keep a lid on the container when not in use.

"Salves can be made out of many herbs using this recipe," says Kirsten. "A good drawing herb would be 1 part plantain and 1 part comfrey. Chickweed and comfrey make a good baby salve for rashes. You

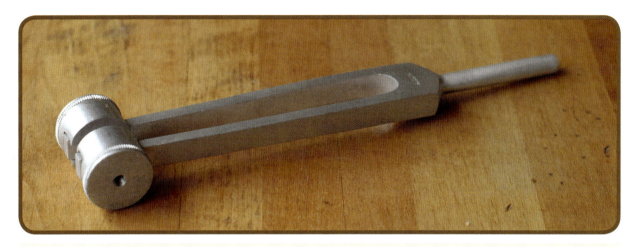

You can use a tuning fork to reveal whether a bone is broken. The weights on the end of the tines help the fork to vibrate longer.

can personalize your salves by deciding which herbs would benefit you and then dividing up the total amount of herb needed. It is a great way to explore your creativity!"

This salve will keep for a long time. If the salve begins to smell rancid, throw it out and make a fresh salve.

TUNING FORKS FOR BROKEN BONES

When you need to find out if a bone is broken, get a tuning fork going and stick it on the area you suspect might be broken.

"If they scream, it is broken," says Kirsten with a laugh.

Even modern podiatrists use tuning forks to determine whether small bones inside the foot are broken. Caleb's own podiatrist regularly uses a tuning fork for this purpose. You can purchase weighted tuning forks that keep the vibration going longer, making the tool easier to use. It is important to

know that the tuning fork must be directly over the break in the bone—Caleb's experiments on people with medically diagnosed broken bones have shown that sometimes if the tuning fork is even a quarter inch to the side of the break, the person will not feel the vibrations of the tuning fork. But if you put the vibrating fork directly over the break, the person will feel an uncomfortable sensation. Because of this, it is important to be thorough when using a tuning fork to reveal whether a bone is broken. Make sure you carefully place the handle of the vibrating fork all over the area where you suspect there might be a break.

At Caleb's house, with small children around, the tuning fork has been a special source of comfort and has been used on many occasions, saving at least hundreds of dollars in medical costs and huge amounts of stress. One example: One day Caleb and his grandson, Xander, were working in the pasture with other family members to install a new fence. Caleb asked six-year-old Xander to run and grab something for him, and Xander took off jogging through some tall weeds, stepping on a rake that had been left lying on the ground. With a loud pop, the handle of the rake jumped up and smacked Xander so hard on the arm that it knocked him over, and he immediately began screaming in serious pain. Caleb was sure that Xander's wrist or forearm had been broken, but the tuning fork revealed no permanent damage, and fifteen agonizing minutes later, Xander was calm once again. Had Kirsten not taught Caleb's family about how to use a tuning fork to diagnose a broken bone, Caleb and the rest of the family would have rushed Xander to the emergency room. X-rays would have revealed that the bone was not broken, and Caleb's family would likely have been left with a not-insignificant bill. Instead, Caleb used the tuning fork, and before long, everyone was working on the fence again—even Xander. This is just one example of the times that children have fallen off of things or jumped off something or otherwise hurt themselves where Caleb's family has been able to use a tuning fork for immediate peace of mind. (This story is also a good example of why tools like rakes should never be left lying on the ground!)

How to Use a Tuning Fork

A tuning fork is actually a musical, not a medical, instrument and can be purchased at any music store. Tuning forks give off a certain tone that musicians use to tune their instruments.

A tuning fork has a handle on one end and two thick tines on the other, forming a narrow U shape. To "start" a tuning fork, you simply pick up the fork by the handle and tap one of the tines against something. You can then place any part of the tuning fork—even the handle—on the area of the body where you suspect there might be a broken bone under the unbroken skin. (Obviously, if a broken bone is protruding from the skin, you don't need a tuning fork—you need emergency medical help.) The vibrating tines cause the broken bone to vibrate against itself, causing a sudden sharp sensation. If a bone is broken, it will be obvious because the person will cry out or try to jerk away from the fork, or both. The tines must be vibrating while touching the skin, or the fork will not work. If you have a brave friend or family member, you can do as Caleb has done and test your tuning fork skills on their broken bone. The pain is momentary and not sharp enough to be intolerable—and ends immediately when the tuning fork is no longer touching the person's skin.

Where to get a tuning fork

Music stores sell tuning forks made for tuning instruments, which do not have weights on the tines. These forks will work, but the vibration does not last long and you may find yourself repeatedly "starting" the fork while trying to diagnose a bone. Weighted tuning forks look exactly like musical tuning forks, except they have one circular weight attached to each tine of the fork. You can purchase these online at amazon.com, for example, or many medical supply stores.

NOTES

1.   John R. Christopher, *School of Natural Healing* (Springville, UT: Christopher Publications, 2010).

CHAPTER 16
HERBS FOR ALLERGIES, BITES, AND STINGS

STINGING NETTLE

Urtica dioica

"Stinging nettle is used copiously in our family for allergies," says Kirsten. "Amazingly enough, the benefit of stinging nettle is its anti-inflammatory property, which at first may seem a little backwards, especially if you have ever been stung by this herb. Made into a tincture using any of the three tincture recipes in this book, nettle is one of the first things our family reaches for when allergy and hay fever season begins. My sister cannot keep enough of it on hand. It alleviates the symptoms associated with allergies in a very short time. We usually take a dropperful at a time for adults and half of that for children. It can be made into a cream for aches and pains as well (recipe below). There is a caution here, however. Because of the anti-inflammatory properties of stinging nettle, and the possibility of it altering the blood system, consult your physician before using nettle if you are pregnant.

"Nettle is also a delicious vegetable, once boiled. I usually gather this with gloves, or grab the stem from the bottom near the soil. It is a beautiful plant that grows near water sources. If stung, look for plantain or burdock to help alleviate the sting—there should be some nearby."

COMMON PLANTAIN

Plantago major

For stings and bites, use common plantain. Plantain is known to herbalists as a drawing plant, similar to onions or mud that is allowed to dry. To use, simply mash fresh plantain leaves and apply them to the sting or bite. If you don't have fresh herb, you can add water to dried plantain.

During a medicinal herb class that Kirsten taught at Caleb's home, one student told a story about her husband, a landscaper, who was working on a nearby mountainside when he was bitten by a hornet. Using

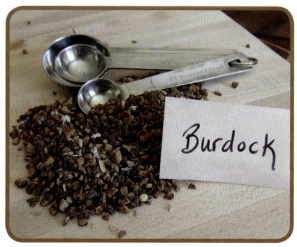

his cell phone, he called his wife and asked her what to do. Over the phone, she guided him to find a plantain plant only steps away, and then instructed him to chew up the leaves and apply them to the sting. His pain went away instantly and he continued his work for the rest of the day. Caleb and Kirsten have both had similar experiences. Plantain is an especially useful remedy if you are outside with children at home or at a park or an event and they get bitten or stung.

"Our world is organized in an amazing way," Kirsten says. "Opposites grow near each other. For instance, when I went on a hike with my family, my niece rubbed against nettle. I looked around for a moment and found some burdock. I squashed the leaves and applied the poultice. The stinging was alleviated."

Using fresh herbs straight from the ground in an emergency is also a good way to introduce the power of herbal medicine to those around you. When trying to help other people understand natural healing, we have to accept people where they are. Many people will look at you suspiciously if you even mention natural medicine—they will assume you have joined a multi-level marketing company and you

want them to join your "sales downline." Or if you try to use herbal treatments on people around you, even your spouse or children—sometimes especially your spouse or children—they will shy away, thinking you've been spending too much time on Facebook or the internet. Perhaps nothing opens people to possibilities like pain, and if you grab a leaf and mash it, promising instant relief, most people will take you up on your offer. This can be the beginning of something beautiful—the sting will go away, leaving behind clear evidence that herbs have medicinal power, if you know how and when to use them.

HIVES

Hives can be treated by drinking nettle tincture or nettle tea.

SNAKEBITE

While we recommend seeking immediate medical attention in the case of snakebite, medical attention is not always immediately available. If you

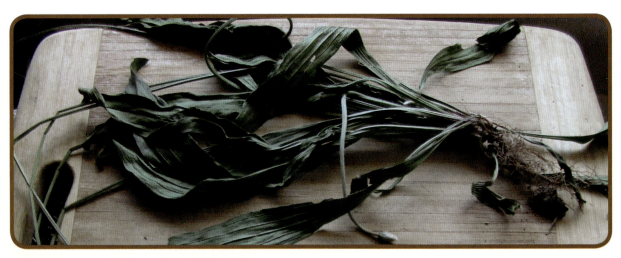

Plantain leaves can be used to draw out poison.

have no other option, echinacea (also called purple coneflower; scientific name *Echinacea purpurea*) contains hyaluronic acid, which both historical and modern evidence says helps treat animal bites and even gunshot wounds. "This beneficial effect is at least partially explained by many studies showing an inhibition of the enzyme hyaluronidase by polysaccharide and alkylamide fractions from echinacea root extracts," according to a research paper by Wendell Combest, PhD associate professor of Pharmacology at Campbell University in North Carolina. "By preventing the breakdown of this 'cellular cement,' invading microorganisms are prevented from spreading throughout the tissue... Several clinical studies have been reported demonstrating echinacea's wound-healing effects. The largest study involved 4,598 patients treated with a salve made from Echinacea purpurea leaves and flowers."[1]

Kirsten suggests using a whole bottle of echinacea tincture in case of snake bite. If tincture is not available, chew and swallow the leaves, flower petals, or roots, and apply chewed leaves of plantain to the wound area, followed by chewed leaves of echinacea.

TREATING SPIDER BITES

Draw out the poison with mashed plantain leaves, and then treat the wound with echinacea tincture both internally and externally.

MANAGING PAIN WITH HERBS

No one wants to live with pain, especially not in today's modern world. Nowhere is this more evident than in sales of over-the-counter pain medications.

Acetaminophen, which is the scientific name for generic Tylenol, might well be the most popular legal drug in the world. It is also an example of the failure of the government and the corporate world to protect human health in the face of huge profits.[2]

Tylenol was introduced to the world in 1955 by McNeil Laboratories of Philadelphia. It was the first aspirin-free pain reliever. In 1959, Tylenol was approved for sale without a prescription. Today, even as Tylenol has become a large line of products, it has also become the number one bestselling over-the-counter analgesic pain reliever in the world—with sales of over $1 billion a year.[3]

Tylenol has been a wonder drug to many, including Caleb. But the public has been shocked to learn, on several occasions, that Tylenol might not be as safe as we thought.

"Acetaminophen overdose is the leading cause for calls to Poison Control Centers (>100,000/year) and accounts for more than 56,000 emergency room visits, 2,600 hospitalizations, and an estimated 458 deaths due to acute liver failure each year," according to a summary of the outcome of the U.S. Acute Liver Failure Study Group. "Available in many single or combination products, acetaminophen produces more than 1 billion US dollars in annual sales for Tylenol products alone. It is heavily marketed for its safety compared to nonsteroidal analgesics. By enabling self-diagnosis and treatment of minor aches and pains, its benefits are said by the Food and Drug Administration to outweigh its risks. It still must be asked: Is this amount of injury and death really acceptable for an over-the-counter pain reliever?"[4]

"Because of continued reports of liver injury, FDA proposes that boxed warnings, the agency's strongest warning for prescription drugs, be added to all acetaminophen prescription products," said the U.S. Food and Drug Administration in a statement in 2011. "Most of the cases of severe liver injury occurred in patients who took more than the prescribed dose of an acetaminophen-containing product in a 24-hour period, took more than one acetaminophen-containing product at the same time, or drank alcohol while taking acetaminophen products."[5]

Companies producing acetaminophen products were asked, but not required, to lower the dose of the drug in their products. Three years later, in 2014, the FDA issued a new statement saying that only "more than half" of companies had complied with their request. "In the near future we intend to institute proceedings to withdraw approval of prescription combination drug products containing more than 325 mg of acetaminophen per dosage unit that remain on the market," said FDA officials in January 2014.[6]

The astonishing thing about all of this is that acetaminophen had been on the market with every possible approval for 59 years when the FDA issued its warning in 2014.

At one point, before Caleb and his family had begun to move toward natural medicine, his wife became alarmed at the amounts of this pain reliever he was taking. Back in the days before Caleb used natural medicine to get his sinus infections under control, two doctors warned Caleb that he had already exceeded the amount needed to begin damaging his liver. Both doctors ordered Caleb to stop.

"I didn't," says Caleb.

Why? He was in pain, and didn't know he had other options. What a relief—literally—when Kirsten introduced Caleb to willow bark and mullein.

WILLOW BARK

Scientific names: Willow family (the bark can be up to 12 percent medicinal)

- White willow/European willow (*Salix alba*)
- Black willow/pussy willow (*Salix nigra*)
- Crack willow (*Salix fragilis*)
- Purple willow (*Salix purpurea*)
- Weeping willow (*Salix babylonica*)[7]

The opinion of modern science about willow bark is a fascinating study in the ongoing tension between natural medicine and the so-called "science" needed for even the simplest drug, used for millennia, to win modern "approval" from government and big business.[8]

"Willow bark is the bark from several varieties of the willow tree, including white willow or European willow, black willow or pussy willow, crack willow, purple willow, and others," according to Webmd.com. "The bark is used to make medicine. Willow bark acts a lot like aspirin, so it is used for pain, including headache, muscle pain, menstrual cramps, rheumatoid arthritis, osteoarthritis, gout, and a disease of the spine called ankylosing spondylitis."

We use Webmd.com's description here because it is telling of the attitude of modern medicine toward all things natural and herbal. Here is what WebMD has to say next about willow bark:

"Willow bark's pain relieving potential has been recognized throughout history. Willow bark was commonly used during the time of Hippocrates, when people were advised to chew on the bark to relieve pain and fever. Willow bark is also used for fever, the common cold, flu, and weight loss... Willow bark contains a chemical called salicin that is similar to aspirin."

So with this weight of history, surely WebMD will acknowledge that willow bark works, right?

Wrong.

According to WebMD there is "insufficient evidence" that willow bark has any power to treat pain relief for headaches, fever, joint pain, arthritis and more. WebMD concludes with this: "More evidence is needed to rate the effectiveness of willow bark for these uses."

Um…

Despite pain relief "recognized throughout history," modern medicine is still on the fence about whether or not willow bark works. Why? What possible evidence could still be needed? Apparently millions of dollars of clinical tests. Those of us who have used willow bark over and over again successfully can only shake our heads and wonder how we will ever survive without the "approval" of the government and big business.

To be fair, not everyone in the medical community refuses to recognize the obvious pain-relieving power of willow bark.

"Willow bark is used to ease pain and reduce inflammation," according to the University of Maryland Medical Center. "Researchers believe that the chemical salicin, found in willow bark, is responsible for these effects. However, studies show several other components of willow bark, including plant chemicals called polyphenols and flavonoids, have antioxidant, fever-reducing, antiseptic, and immune-boosting properties. Some studies show willow is as effective as aspirin for reducing pain and inflammation (but not fever), and at a much lower dose. Scientists think that may be due to other compounds in the herb. More research is needed… In the 1800s, salicin was used to develop aspirin. White willow appears to bring pain relief more slowly than aspirin, but its effects may last longer."[9]

How to Use Willow Bark

Willow bark can be used as a tea or tincture, or you can do as people have done throughout history, and simply chew on the inner bark of the tree.

COMMON MULLEIN

Verbascum thapsus

Sometimes called a torch plant or candlestick plant, mullein has pain-relieving power along with anti-inflammatory power. This beautiful plant grows on mountain hillsides all over the western United States and is often found along the sides of mountain roads in late summer with its four-foot-high single stem of yellow flowers. It is a beautiful, showy biennial plant that Caleb grows in his garden. The leaves are harvested for medicinal use when the plant blooms in the second year.

Tincture of mullein serves as a wonderful substitute for Nyquil or other syrups to help you sleep

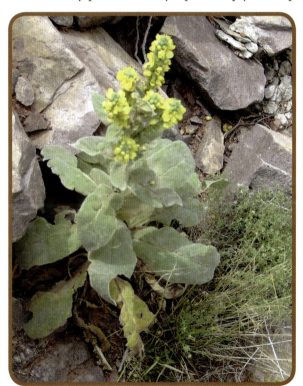

A wild mullein plant in flower. Mullein flower spikes can grow to be five feet tall.

and decongest when you are sick. Caleb takes a tablespoon of the tincture in a glass of warm water before going to bed if he is congested or has sinus pain that keeps him awake.

Mullein tincture can also be applied inside and outside the ear for earache.

Because mullein is a powerful mucus-buster and stimulates the respiratory system, it is used to treat bronchitis and any congestion or trouble breathing.

"Mullein is also for your lymph glands," says Kirsten. "When you have swollen glands, you can take mullein tea. You can also soak a cloth in the mullein tea and wrap it around your neck to treat your glands. This is called a fomentation. Let it sit on your glands until it gets cold, and then do it again."

Mullein Tincture

Mullein must be initially tinctured in alcohol, according to both the authors' experience and the National Formulary of 1888. The medicine of some herbs simple does not release well into any other solution than alcohol, and mullein is one of those. You can remove the alcohol after the mullein is "solved" in solution by following the directions in the Tinctures chapter of this book.

NOTES

1. Wendell Combest and George Nemecz, "Echinacea," *U.S. Pharmacist*, accessed October 21, 2014, http://web.campbell.edu/faculty/nemecz/George_home/references/Echinacea.html.

2. Lee W. M., "Acetaminophen and the U.S. Acute Liver Failure Study Group: Lowering the Risks of Hepatic Failure," *Hepatology* 40, no. 1 (2004): 6–9.

3. "Our Story," Tylenol, accessed October 21, 2014, http://www.tylenol.com/news/about-us.

4. Ibid.

5. "FDA limits acetaminophen in prescription combination products; requires liver toxicity warnings," FDA, last updated January 13, 2011, accessed October 21, 2014, http://www.fda.gov/NewsEvents/Newsroom/PressAnnouncements/ucm239894.htm.

6. "FDA recommends health care professionals discontinue prescribing and dispensing prescription combination drug products with more than 325 mg of acetaminophen to protect consumers," FDA, last updated January 15, 2014, accessed October 21, 2014, http://www.fda.gov/Drugs/DrugSafety/ucm381644.htm.

7. "Willow Bark," University of Maryland Medical Center, accessed October 21, 2014, http://umm.edu/health/medical/altmed/herb/willow-bark#ixzz2yX1f9Zo0.

8. "Willow Bark," WebMD, accessed October 21, 2014, http://www.webmd.com/vitamins-supplements/ingredientmono-955-WILLOW%20BARK.aspx?activeIngredientId=955&activeIngredientName=WILLOW%20BARK.

9. "Willow Bark," University of Maryland Medical Center, Accessed October 21, 2014, http://umm.edu/health/medical/altmed/herb/willow-bark#ixzz2yX1f9Zo0.

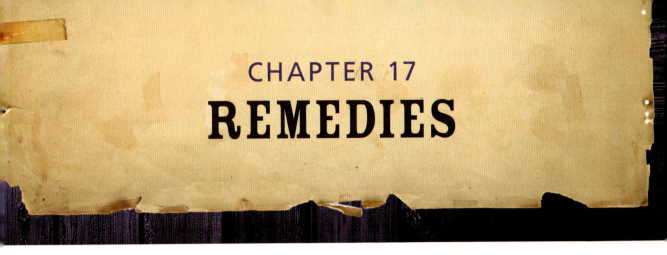

CHAPTER 17
REMEDIES

SINUS RINSING

When it comes to saving yourself, there is perhaps nothing more simple and powerful than the age-old practice of sinus rinsing. Salt water is used to rinse out the sinus, washing away allergens, dust, pollen, mucus, bacteria, viruses, and any other foreign matter that is collected in the sinus cavity. *Collected* is an apropos word here—the sinus is designed to be the body's air filtration system. The sinus, working with the hairs in our noses, literally captures the tiny things we breathe, encasing them in mucus so they can be expelled. Overloading the system, however, often leads to inflammation in the sinus. Inflammation is the body's way of capturing and isolating foreign matter in mucus in an attempt to remove it from the body. Unfortunately, infection can set in.

Sinus rinsing changed Caleb's life, and the more you learn about this, the more you will hear the words "changed my life." Many, many people who have suffered from chronic sinusitis or allergies for years have found permanent, drug-free, chemical-free, steroid-free relief by simply rinsing their sinus with saline. You simply squeeze saline into one nostril, and it immediately flows through the sinus cavity and drains out the other nostril.

When Caleb first started sinus rinsing, it was lesser known and not as popular, but today sinus rinsing kits can now be found at most grocery stores and almost all pharmacies. There are two kinds—squeeze bottles and neti pots. Neti pots require you to pour the water into your sinus. Squeeze bottles allow you to gently squeeze water into the sinus. Both work, but the squeeze bottle is much easier to use. Caleb uses a NeilMed plastic squeeze bottle that can be sanitized in boiling water as often as wanted.

NeilMed, which brought sinus rinsing to the masses in the United States, sells prepackaged

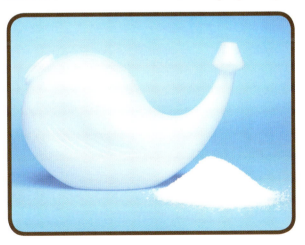

A neti pot is used for nasal irrigation.

pulverized salt packs that are pre-measured and inexpensive. They also sell a special package that is a combination of salt and baking soda. The goal of sinus rinsing is to prevent allergies and infections, and for daily maintenance, salt water is perfect. However, if you have any kind of swelling, tightness, or drainage, use the salt-baking soda combo, which is a powerful way to cut mucus. The baking soda combination can sting slightly, but it is well worth it. Caleb, who has suffered a lifetime of sinusitis, will take the momentary stinging sensation over a sinus infection any day!

Recipe for Sinus Rinsing

- 1 cup warm water (not hot)
- ½ teaspoon pulverized sea salt (NOT iodized table salt)
- ¼ teaspoon baking soda (optional)

STEP 1. Mix water and salt (and soda, if needed) in water. Dissolve completely.

STEP 2. Using a commercial squeeze bottle, squeeze gently (not fast, not hard) into one nostril while in the shower or standing over the bathroom sink. The rinse will immediately come out the other nostril. When your rinse bottle is empty, turn your head first to one side and then the other while gently blowing out air. This helps get out all the saline solution.

STEP 3. Repeat as often as necessary. For maintenance, once a day or as needed is common. If someone in your home or at your work is sick, rinse several times a day. If you are sick, you can rinse as often as you want, even hourly.

DEPRESSION

Depression is a wide topic that can range from garden-variety sadness and grief all the way to brain disorders like post-traumatic stress disorder. Struggles with crippling depression are highly individual, and so are the treatments. There is no "one size fits all" answer to depression, but there are some natural remedies and herbs that have a proven history of being useful in treating depression.

There are numerous small things anyone can do to help manage depression, starting with eating a healthy diet. Kirsten suggests trying the simple step of electrical grounding.

"We are electrical beings," says Kirsten. "It is important that we are grounded by being barefoot on the earth. I once cleared the snow off the grass and walked on it in winter after my doctor told me to, and it helped."

Physical touch also has the power to lift our spirits, so don't be afraid to ask for a hug, or give a hug, if you need to. Tell whomever you are hugging that you read in a wonderful book that you need to hug more people, more often!

Yoga has some power to relieve depression, as does any form of exercise. Having a pet can help. Some people swear by meditation. Learning to play a Tibetan singing bowl is easy, fun, and seems to have some real sway over the dark cloud of depression. Small Tibetan singing bowls are inexpensive to order online, and with a little practice you feel almost magic as you learn to make the bowl sing. Singing bowls are often added to meditation routines, and can be pulled out any time depression weighs you down.

St. John's wort is a powerful herb with a long history of use to combat depression both historically and today. St. John's wort is best used in a glycerin tincture, using the recipe in this book.

"Though I support herbal remedies for depression, there are times when the mental health or life of a person outweighs the side effects of prescription medication," says Kirsten. "Make your decisions wisely. And a word of warning: Those who are currently taking antidepressants should not stop or reduce their medication in favor of St. John's wort or any other alternative remedy without the assistance of their physician."

TREATING BURNS

"Don't use salves on burns because salves contain wax," says Kirsten. "Instead, use honey burn paste, which is antibacterial. For the past 10 years, I have had the opportunity to be a volunteer and employee at This Is The Place Heritage Park. It is a living historical village nestled in a corner of the Salt Lake Valley. I had the opportunity of working in the Anderson home, where we demonstrated how to cook on a wood stove and offered the guests delicious treats. One day, the young woman I was working with burned her hand on the wood stove. I asked her if I could help her and she said yes. I then went down the lane and collected several fresh comfrey leaves that were planted for their beauty. Bringing them back, I crushed some of the leaves and showed her how to apply them to the wound. She continued to add freshly crushed comfrey as the leaves dried and was healed within a few hours. My oldest son, Garrett, was an apprentice to the blacksmith at the same park. I had him keep some comfrey salve in his possession due to the flying sparks as the metal was heated and shaped. Comfrey is wonderful as a burn cream. According to Dr. Christopher, the comfrey should be combined with honey, an antibiotic, and wheat germ oil, which is known to heal skin without scars. You can mix it as needed ⅓ of each by volume. It is best made fresh."

Honey Burn Paste

- 1 part comfrey (fresh or dried)
- 1 part honey
- 1 part wheat germ oil

STEP 1. Mix ingredients. Always make this paste fresh when you need it. Do not make ahead and store.

STEP 2. Apply the paste to the burn and wrap the wounded area with gauze. Over time, the paste will disappear as it is absorbed into the body. When it is gone, make a fresh batch of paste and put it on again, at least once a day. Continue this until the burn is healed.

HERBS FOR KIDNEY HEALTH

To encourage kidney health, use:

- Parsley tea or tincture
- Uva ursi herb tea or tincture
- Cramp bark tea or tincture
- Juniper berry tincture
- Lobelia tea or tincture
- Enuresis, also called incontinence, is the inability to control the bladder at night. There are several herbal options to help treat this in adults and children. Parsley tea in the morning will help children avoid wetting the bed at night.

HERBS FOR CALMING & SOOTHING NERVES

"I think that everyone has their favorite stress reliever, also called a nervine," says Kirsten. "There are several nervines, also called antispasmodics. I usually keep several on hand including skullcap, valerian, lobelia, catnip, and lemon balm. The first three I keep in tinctures and the last two I like to have fresh. When I feel stressed, I take one of these tinctures or teas. I prefer to use skullcap with children and rub it on the base of their neck and down the spine. It is immediately relaxing. Valerian is very strong and can have the opposite effect on some people. Mentioning several of them is beneficial because some are more readily available to one person than another."

- Catnip (also called *catnep* or *catmint*) is used for children because of its mild flavor and reaction.

- Lemon balm, which is also called melissa, with its bright lemon scent "smells the best to me, and sometimes that is all that is required," says Kirsten.

- Skullcap works best with those children who have a very erratic temperament and need their whole body to become calm as soon as possible in order to function. Tincture of skullcap can be rubbed up and down the spine to create calming in a person.

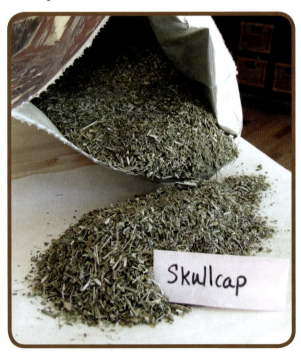

Dried skullcap plant ready for homemade use.

- Tincture of lobelia acts as a sedative when combined with another nervine such as skullcap, lemon balm, or catnip.

ATHLETE'S FOOT

- Use black walnut tincture to rub on feet to treat athlete's foot and air-dry. A salve may be preferable.

- Add Epsom salts to a warm foot bath.

- Put black walnut powder in your sock.

ANTIBIOTIC

Powder of goldenseal root is a powerful antibiotic that can be added to tea or made into a tincture. "Whether or not this is recommendable I don't know, but when I have a bad sinus infection, I inhale a quarter-teaspoon of goldenseal root powder straight up my nostril," says Caleb. "It helps immensely, immediately acting to help break up the mucus, fight the infection, and clear my sinus. If the infection has a strong hold, I will do this every several hours— I will do just about anything to avoid the crippling migraine that my sinus infections always seem to end in."

COUGHS, COLDS, FLU, AND INFLAMMATION

When anyone is suffering for a respiratory illness, there is a mantra that saves lives:

"Dry and hot = Death."

What this means is that the key to treating respiratory illness is to keep the body hydrated, which in turn allows the body to keep the mucus moving and

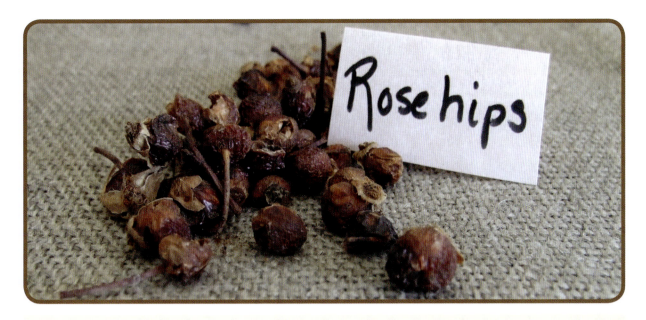

Rosehips are rich in natural vitamin C, which is an important immune system stimulant

fight the infection. Mucus clogs the flow of toxins exiting the body, so it is important to help the body expel mucus. The importance of keeping the mucus moving cannot be overstated! There are several things we can do to help our bodies perform our task.

"We can use hot baths to sweat out toxins," says Kirsten. "We can make sure our bowels are functioning properly to allow the release of mucus and toxins. We can vomit, or expel mucus through our sinuses."

Bowel cleansers include the herbs senna leaf, cascara sagrada, and turkey rhubarb, among others. It is important to note that each of these herbs has a specific purpose and works at different intensities. Senna leaf is very powerful; it acts on the entire intestinal area. Be aware that taking senna will definitely do the job for those who are constipated, and it will do that job for several hours. There may be cramping involved. Cascara sagrada can be mild or as powerful as senna depending on the amount used. It strengthens the entire elimination tract and the organs that

are involved. Because it is used to strengthen, it is used usually used as part of a regular or daily healing routine. Turkey rhubarb helps the muscles of the lower bowel to work more effectively. It is a good herb for children, taken in small doses. Be aware that larger amounts can cause cramping.

Keeping your bowels clean is one of the most important principles of healthy living. Most disease is related to how well we eliminate. Though it is sometimes embarrassing to discuss, it must be done. The first thing I ask my family when they are sick is, "Have you gone to the bathroom lately?" Then I drill them. How much? how often? how big? what color? what consistency? Think of our canine friends. If they eat twice per day, how many times do you need to pick up after them? Twice. If you eat 3–4 times per day, how often should you be eliminating? If we are not eliminating, we are causing a backup in the very system that is meant to keep us healthy and clean. Toxins are part of our environment and they will cause illness.

Vomiting is cleansing. We eliminate unwanted elements from our body through our sweat, our nose, bowel movements, vomiting, and spitting. However, vomiting can cause dehydration, which can be dangerous. As explained in another chapter, lobelia can be used to stop vomiting if needed.

Colds

- Echinacea helps us build up our immune system.

- Rosehips and pine needle tea are both rich in natural vitamin C, which is an important immune system stimulant.

- Add cayenne to your daily treatment.

- Horseradish steam vapor. Place crushed horseradish root in steaming water and inhale the vapors by placing a towel over your head as you breathe in over the bowl.

- Yarrow is a diaphoretic, which means it makes you sweat and breaks up congestion and fevers. Yarrow has been successfully used by the Native Americans, pioneers and settlers, and herbalists of today and yesterday.

Homemade Cough Syrup Recipe

- 1 finely chopped medium onion

- honey

STEP 1. Put the chopped onion in a pan and coat it with honey until the onion is covered. Cook for 20 minutes on low heat. Do not boil.

STEP 2. Strain the onion out of the honey and bottle the honey. This keeps a long time. You can add black cherry tincture before you bottle it.

OPTIONAL: You can add ¼ cup black cherry bark and ½ cup dried mullein to the onion mash when you cook it. These ingredients will make it more effective, but if you don't have them, don't be afraid to just make the onion honey syrup.

Bronchitis Treatments

- Onion poultice, as outlined in the The Common Onion chapter of this book.

- Mullein tincture for pain and respiratory easing.

- Eat slippery elm gruel. Slippery elm gruel is a mucilaginous herb. It soothes the tissues of the digestive tract. It is slightly sweet and it goes down very easily. It is safe for children and

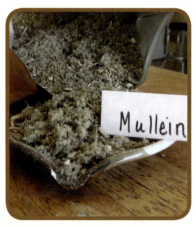

Dried mullein for making tinctures

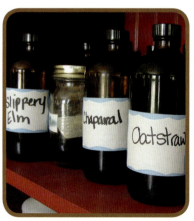

Tinctures are kept in dark bottles while storing.

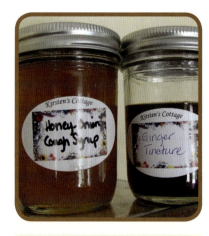

Cough syrup and ginger tincture

adults. Taken in larger amounts throughout the day, it can help expel mucus as well. Some take it in capsules, though I think the soothing properties of the herb have more benefit on the throat and esophagus when taken as gruel. It should be accompanied with adequate drinking water. As always, if you are pregnant, consult a doctor before taking any herbal supplements.

Slippery Elm Gruel Recipe

- 2 generous tablespoons of dried slippery elm

- ¾ cup warm water

STEP 1. Mix dried herb and water. Let it sit for a moment until it thickens somewhat.

STEP 2. (optional) Mix in applesauce and a bit of cinnamon. More water can be added as desired.

- Mustard seed plaster. Please note that this is not the condiment mustard in your kitchen. Mustard seed can be found at the health food store.

Mustard Plaster Recipe

- ¼ cup mustard seed powder

- 1 cup flour

- Wheat germ oil, enough to make a cream or plaster.

STEP 1. Mix ingredients.

STEP 2. Put the plaster on a cloth and apply the cloth to the chest.

Sore Throat

- Licorice tea. Please note that medicinal licorice is an herb, not a candy. It's scientific name is *Glycyrrhiza glabra*. For information, visit SeedRenaissance.com and click on "Apothecary." Licorice tea is good for the glandular system.

- Lemon tea.

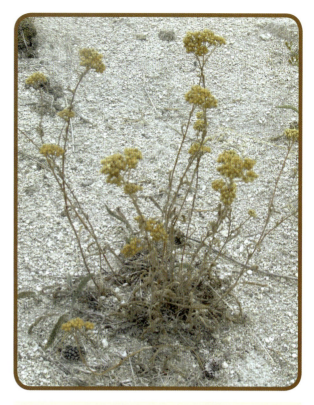

Yarrow at Yellowstone National Park, dry and yellow in late autumn (too late for fresh harvesting).

- Horehound tea, tincture, lozenge, or old-fashioned hard candy. This is used as an expectorant and to ease congestion. Caleb prefers horehound from his garden in a warm tea for congestion. "As a fun sidenote, the ancient Egyptian priests honored its medicinal properties and its ability to break magic spells," says Kirsten.

NAUSEA

- Red raspberry tea with a few drops of lobelia tincture.

- Ginger root powder with baking soda and water, ginger works better than Dramamine for

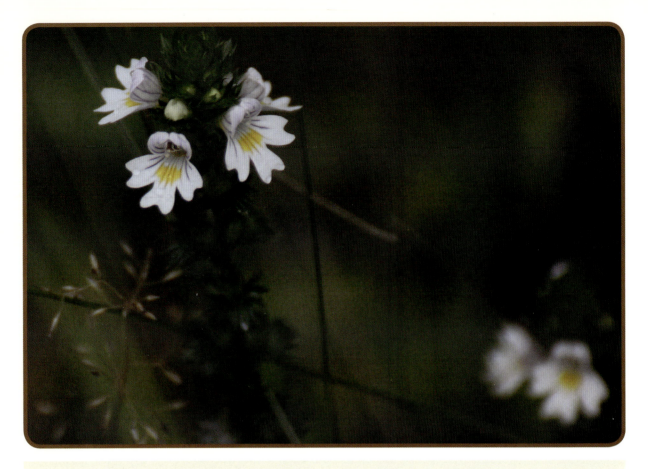

Eyebright, also called Euphrasia, is named for its ability to treat eye infections

motion sickness etc. (1 teaspoon ginger root, dash of baking soda, 1 cup warm water).

• Peppermint tea.

GROWING PAINS

When Caleb was a teen, he suffered from terrible growing pains—horrible cramps in his legs at night that felt like they would snap his bones. Decades later, he still gets leg cramps occasionally. To help relieve this pain, Kirsten suggests cramp bark (*Viburnum opulus*), which is a relaxant and antispasmodic.

"Though normally used in tincture form to relax the uterus and ovaries, it can relax all kinds of nerves and muscle spasms," she says. "It is also a sedative, which would help children relax and sleep. Children who suffer from growing pains may benefit from the use of cramp bark. I have never had the opportunity to use this myself, but the evidence supports this finding."

HERBS FOR THE EYES

Spend much time on the computer? You can relieve eyestrain instantly with the herb eyebright.

Make eyebright tea and apply it directly onto your eyeballs using a glass eyeball cup, which you can get at health food stores, herb shops, or online. You can also find beautiful eyewash cups at antique stores. Fill the cup with eyebright tea, put your eye to the cup, and then blink into the tea, washing the eyeball. Kirsten also makes an herbal eyewash.

Herbal Eyewash Recipe

- 1 tablespoon eyebright
- 1 cup of water
- ½ teaspoon goldenseal
- ½ teaspoon bayberry
- ¼ teaspoon cayenne

STEP 1. Make a tea from the ingredients and strain.

STEP 2. Put mixture into eyewash cup and apply to eyeball as a wash.

NOTE: You may have to work up to this amount of cayenne. If you are new to cayenne, start with one drop instead of a quarter-teaspoon.

TO COMBAT ABDOMINAL GAS

- Peppermint tincture or tea before or after a meal.
- Fennel tincture or tea before or after a meal.
- You can also eat charcoal, which is a favorite of Kirsten's husband. Please note, charcoal does not mean the briquettes from a bag that you use for backyard grilling. This is campfire charcoal. You can eat a teaspoon or tablespoon at most. Never eat charcoal that is hot—it should be completely cooled, "dead" charcoal. Be aware of your source of charcoal; only wood charcoal should be used.

FOR NATURAL VITAMIN C

- Wild rosehips. These can be gathered from spent roses in your backyard in autumn or winter. Peel off and eat the leathery outer cover.
- White pine needle is also an excellent source of vitamin C.

HEART HEALTH

- Brigham Tea can be used as an everyday tonic. It has natural ephedra in it, so it stimulates the heart and is slightly drying, which helps with the build-up of mucus. Use Brigham Tea when the leafstick is black in the middle—it is a plant of sticks with no leaves.
- The herb chaparral, used as a tea or tincture, is a blood cleanser

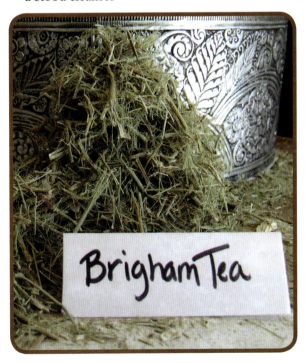

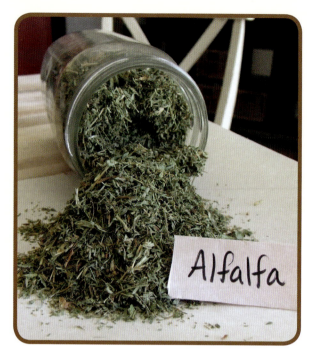
Alfalfa

- Hawthorn berry tincture is excellent for heart health.

- Cayenne in Shock Tea, as mentioned in the Cayenne chapter of this book, will stimulate the heart.

- Apple cider vinegar with honey in water is a good artery cleanser.

BACTERIA AND FUNGUS

Myrrh is Kirsten's favorite herb for fighting bacteria and fungus. There has been research conducted at Rutgers University and the University of Cairo in Egypt that indicates it has a positive effect in fighting cancer.[1]

These studies show that myrrh kills the cancer cells without killing the healthy cells. These studies suggest more research is needed to pursue myrrh as a cancer treatment. As an herbalist, it shows that

answers do exist to our most difficult questions, if we know where to look. Myrrh was one of the three gifts given to Jesus Christ by the wise men that visited him as a child. Maybe there is more wisdom here than just the traditional title.

MAYBE KIDS SHOULD EAT DIRT

Studies show that our children's immune systems are weaker than the generations previous because they are not exposed to enough low levels of inoculating germs found naturally in dirt. In a January 26, 2009, *New York Times* article titled "Babies Know: A Little Dirt Is Good for You,"[2] writer Jane Brody says that clinical studies "strongly" suggest that bacteria, viruses, and especially worms in dirt help kids development a healthy immune system. "Several continuing studies suggest that worms may help to redirect an immune system that has gone awry and resulted in autoimmune disorders, allergies, and asthma. These studies, along with epidemiological observations, seem to explain why immune system disorders like multiple sclerosis, Type 1 diabetes, inflammatory bowel disease, asthma, and allergies have risen significantly in the United States and other developed countries," Brody writes. She quotes Dr. Joel V. Weinstock, director of gastroenterology and hepatology at Tufts Medical Center in Boston as saying that public health measures, like cleaning up contaminated water and food, have saved the lives of countless children, but they "also eliminated exposure to many organisms that are probably good for us. Children raised in an ultraclean environment are not being exposed to organisms that help them develop appropriate immune regulatory circuits." For more information, get the book *Why Dirt Is Good* by microbiologist Mary Ruebush.[3]

POWER FOODS

"We are what we eat—this is a phrase that has been used for as long as I can remember," says Kirsten. "It is a good thing this is not literal. There is a definite relationship between what we eat, or don't eat, and our health. All engines require a particular gas, and if you don't have the right gas, you blow the engine. Your body is an amazing engine. And you need the right fuel."

Especially if you are sick, eating a mucus-less diet is probably one of the most important things you can do for your health. That means avoiding food that causes mucus buildup, including dairy, meat, sugar, flour, and processed foods.

"We should also include eating foods with the highest nutritional value and the most enzymes, vegetables, fruit, nuts, seeds, and whole unprocessed grains," says Kirsten. "There are many versions of the perfect eating plan. I am explaining the ideal that I believe will produce the best health. I ate a vegetarian diet for many years. Finding myself hungry and unsatisfied, I chose to incorporate meat into our diet. I still believe in the words of Jack LaLanne: 'If God made it, I will eat it.' He was a proponent of eating his vegetables and staying away from processed foods."

Remember that many herbal remedies incorporate regular food, like onions, garlic, and apple cider vinegar. We should also remember the antibiotic properties of honey (not to be used for babies), the omegas that are a part of nuts and seeds, particularly flax, and the nutritional value of raw olive oil and raw coconut oil.

There are amazing benefits to citrus, including the immune-fighting capabilities of vitamin C.

"I have felt better physically by eating a wide variety of the foods that have been provided for mankind, with a heavy emphasis on vegetables and fruits," says Kirsten. "Herbs are in the vegetable family. Greens of every kind including alfalfa, wild greens like dandelion, and processed greens like wheat grass, followed by ample amounts of pure water, will help speed our bodies on to greater health. Take a look at what is on your plate. Does it have a purpose? Does it benefit your life? In the book *Dinotopia* by James Gurney they have a saying: *Eat to live, don't live to eat.*[4] That is the best advice I have ever encountered."

WATER

- Water is perhaps the most important power food. Drinking more water and less soda and juice will greatly benefit your health. Distilled water will help clean the extra minerals that have

Dandelion greens aid in cleansing the liver

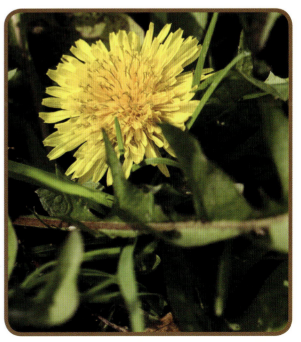

built up in your system because distilled water absorbs minerals. It is also best to use distilled water when making tea for the same reason, because distilled water will pull out the healing properties from the herbs. When making tinctures, always use distilled water.

- Alfalfa leaves in salad or dried and crushed and put in green drinks or tinctures "contain every mineral known to man," says Kirsten.

- Flax contains omega fatty acids, which are oils our bodies need for our brain and organ functions.

- Dandelion greens aid in cleaning the liver.

- Bowel cleansers include the herbs senna leaf, cascara sagrada, and turkey rhubarb.

FIVE EASIEST WAYS TO IMMEDIATELY IMPROVE HEALTH

1. No more soda.

2. Replace sugary cereal with a homemade hot breakfast.

3. As a rule, eat desserts only when made from scratch

4. Learn to cook with stevia instead of sugar.

5. Start practicing the forgotten art of quarantine. If you have a sick person at home, keep everyone else out of the room as much as humanly possible.

NOTES

1. Rebecca Joy Knottnerus, "Myrrh," accessed October 21, 2014, http://www.herballegacy.com/Knottnerus_Medicinal.html.

2. Jane Brody, "Babies Know: A Little Dirt Is Good for You," *New York Times*, Jaunary 26, 2009, accessed October 21, 2014, http://www.nytimes.com/2009/01/27/health/27brod.html?_r=0.

3. Mary Ruebush, *Why Dirt is Good: 5 Ways to Make Germs Your Friends* (Fort Lauderdale, FL: Kaplan, 2009).

4. James Gurney, *Dinotopia: A Land Apart from Time* (Nashville, TN: Turner Publishing, 1994), 77.

CHAPTER 18

CALEB WARNOCK

"THE FORGOTTEN ART OF THE QUARANTINE"

T hey dies everywheres," said the boy. "They dies in their lodgings . . . and they dies . . . in heaps. They dies more than they lives."[1]

On Wednesday, May 8, 2013, my wife found me passed out on the bedroom floor. This is the story of my comeuppance.

I first felt a tickle in my throat on Sunday afternoon, May 5. By this time, my wife had been sick for nine days. A hell-bent virus had swept through our extended family, toppling everyone into bed one by one. I alone was untouched—and I had gotten cocky about it. I had been publicly evangelizing the virtues of sinus rinsing. Twice in the previous month I had given public demonstrations in classes at my home (one woman left the room and wouldn't watch. "No extra charge for that," I quipped when I dripped on another woman's notes and she protested).

My confidence was earned. Sinus rinsing, as you have read in another chapter of this book, had changed my life. By May 5, 2013, I had handily avoided many family illnesses by faithfully rinsing. I had every confidence that this wave of illness would be no different.

When my wife first got sick, she told me to quarantine myself by sleeping in another room of the house. I was so confident in the protective power of nasal rinsing that I dismissed the idea. After nine days of being right, sinus rinsing had become my superpower.

Then the tickle at the back of my throat.

"You had better turn him out," said Mr. Skimpole.
"What do you mean?" inquired my guardian, almost sternly.
"My dear Jarndyce," said Mr. Skimpole, "I have a constitutional objection to this sort of thing. I always had, when I was a medical man. He's not safe, you know. There's a very bad sort of fever about him."[2]

By Wednesday, May 8, I was feverish and aggressively treating myself herbally—using my own blend of marshmallow root, mullein tincture, yarrow flower, and other herbs in tandem with peppermint compresses, rinsing my sinus with salt and sodium bicarbonate, and pounding fresh yarrow leaves from my garden for anti-inflammatory tea. But I worsened.

That morning, I drove myself to the doctor. My

wife's virus had turned into infection in her ear, and I was afraid I might follow. The doctor determined there was no bacterial infestation in me and wrote a prescription for a lidocaine gargle to numb my throat, which by this time felt like it was bleeding.

Driving home, I began to see auras. A migraine caused by sinus swelling and triggered by the sunlight had set in. By early afternoon, and home alone, I was in exquisite pain. I tried to crawl from the bed to the phone to call 911. On the floor, I began to vomit so fast and hard I could not breathe. Then I passed out.

At some point my wife came home and found me on the floor. Rousing me, she listened as I whispered "blessing." She got a member of our lay Mormon clergy—my son-in-law happened to be nearest—who rubbed consecrated olive oil onto the crown of my head before laying his hands on me to give me a blessing by the authority of the holy Melchizedek

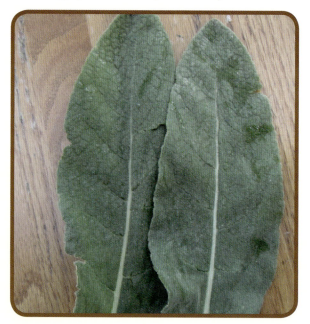

Mullein leaves can be used topically to soften and protect the skin.

priesthood and in the name of Jesus Christ. I then whispered for Excedrin Migraine, a blend of Tylenol and caffeine. Immediately, I either fell asleep or passed out again.

When I woke up, I felt brand new.

It did not last. The pain slowly redoubled, intensifying through the night.

At some point the next day, I doubled the recommended dose of Excedrin Migraine, on top of the Tylenol I had already taken—a dosage I knew would begin to damage my liver. I was desperate. At some point, it became clear to me that I had about two minutes before I would lose consciousness again. I was home alone again. I had to save myself. I prayed, and saw the image of myself opening my grandmother's fridge. When I was a boy on the farm, and I got a rare migraine, my grandmother would treat me with a cold Coke from her fridge. For decades, she kept one Coke on hand as medicine to cure her own rare headaches. I had been raised to never drink caffeinated soda because—as my grandmother and my mother would say—caffeine is medicine and not a recreational drug. Now, a few months past my 40th birthday, I had not had a single caffeinated anything since being treated by my grandmother decades earlier (I don't even drink non-caffeinated soda). I crawled to the phone and dialed my wife, who immediately left her office to buy me a can of Red Bull.

Within minutes of drinking the Red Bull, I began to weep. For the first time in 30 hours, relief.

It took two more cans to stabilize the pain at a tolerable level. My wife drove me to a chiropractor, who said he could drain my sinus. He couldn't. (He easily accepted an $80 fee, however.) Next Charmayne drove me back to the doctor, who injected me with a steroid in one hip and an anti-nausea drug in the other. Infection had now invaded both my sinus and right ear, and I was prescribed the antibiotic Cefdinir, created in a Japanese laboratory and given an oddly Celtic name.

That night was spent on the hardwood oak floor of the living room. Propped with a wadded quilt, I managed to position myself just right so I could sleep face down for a couple of hours.

The next day, I had my third migraine in three days. This time, it only took two Red Bulls to quell my misery to the point where I could open my eyes. My stepdaughter managed to get my laptop iTunes to play Alanis Morrisette's "Jagged Little Pill"[3] album. I needed distraction from three days of lightning strikes to the brain. I fantasized, envisioning an awl that I would carefully insert between the top of my eye and skull, pounding with my palm until I pierced the pain. Wiggling the wooden handle would allow a cloud of steam-pain to whoosh out of my head. There was no blood in my fantasy. Just relief.

In reality, when "Jagged Little Pill" became annoying, I was too weak to reach over and shut it off.

Like the other days, I wrapped my entire head with a huge frozen gel pack. By now, my forehead and eyelids were literally burned red from peppermint compresses, which gave me a tiny palliative.

These next sentences sound masochistic now, but you have to remember I was on my third migraine in three days. My head felt like it would explode from inflammation. I hit myself on the head with my fist and knuckles for over an hour—tapping and banging circles around the expanding pressure under the left side of my forehead—until I had to stop because of the swelling.

"Charley," said I, "are you so cold?"

"I think I am, miss," she replied. "I don't know what it is. I can't hold myself still. I felt so yesterday at about this same time, miss. Don't be uneasy, I think I'm ill."

I heard Ada's voice outside, and I hurried to the door of communication between my room and our pretty sitting-room, and locked it. Just in time, for she tapped at it while my hand was yet upon the key.

Ada called to me to let her in, but I said, "Not now, my dearest. Go away. There's nothing the matter; I will come to you presently." Ah! It was a long, long time before my darling girl and I were companions again.[4]

Ah, yes. My comeuppance.

We approach sickness much more flippantly today than we did in 1853, when Bleak House—Dickens' best novel—was published in 20 installments. In those days, sick people were immediately and strictly locked in a room, quarantined against infecting everyone around them. When fever took over, you became delirious and then—if you were lucky—you lost consciousness, sometimes for days. There were no antibiotics to save you, no Tylenol for pain, no steroid shots in the hip to drain away the inflammation in the skull. If your fever won the day, you woke up and lived. If your fever lost—well, graveyards were busy places.

Today, we act like we have forgotten all this. Because we have.

Recently, the five-year-old living next door broke his leg at some place where parents pay to let their kids jump on a bunch of indoor trampolines. Literally the next day, our grandson Xander was begging us to go to this place. With a touch of righteous anger, my wife explained to him and me (I was standing nearby, so I was guilty) that a hundred years ago, no one would have let their child jump on a trampoline because if you broke your leg, you had a fifty-fifty chance of dying from infection. Parents took the health of their children very seriously because children routinely died. It was not uncommon for half of your children to die. Men married two and three times because their wives died in childbirth. Just this week, there was a major story in our local newspaper about a stunningly beautiful young woman who died in a neighboring town while giving birth to her sixth child. The placenta had attached to her organs and she went into cardiac arrest during a C-section. The baby lived. This happens so very rarely today that it was front-page news. In 1853, it was too common to make headlines.

It was not until Charley was safe in bed again and placidly asleep that I began to think the contagion of her illness was upon me. I had been able easily to hide what I felt at tea-time, but I was past that already now, and I knew that I was rapidly following in Charley's steps.[5]

If we—my wife, me, the kids, the grandkids—had been living in 1853 when this wretched virus mowed us down, how many of us would have lived?

The question is a trick. The answer is that our family would likely have been little scathed, because at the first sign of illness, the sick person would have been quarantined swiftly and strictly. In those days, this was the drill: One "brave" person would be placed in the quarantined room to care for the sick. The sick would become well and then take care of the caretaker, who had now succumbed to the contagion. Daily food and updates were passed through an outside window. The quarantined room was eventually unlocked and—ideally—two people emerged. (The "brave" person assigned to care for the sick was rarely the mother. She was too important. It was usually an older sibling—he or she only had an iffy chance of living to adulthood anyway.)

My family was saved by modern medicine. But we were sickened in the first place by modern stupidity. How I wish now that I had followed my wife's advice and slept in another room! (The only advice my own mother has given me since my wedding day: "Do what your wife says.")

When master herbalist Kirsten Skirvin taught herbal healing classes around my kitchen table, she spoke of earthquakes. If the earth moves violently, we will be on our own because hospitals will either be flattened, or swamped with critical cases. Herbal knowledge may be the only thing we have for our family (Kirsten will be busy, for sure). I would suggest that we will need to add the old art of quarantine to our efforts, if we really want to save lives.

And foolish is the person (ahem—me) who waits until a crisis to remember the virtues of quarantine. Voluntary household quarantine should be used today—without waiting for an earthquake or the zombie apocalypse.

We rely too much on doctors to save us. We are too casual with the health of our youngsters.

When sick, we are far too quick to go to church and school, fanning our disease across town. We have been medically spoiled—may our lives always be so. But a pinch of quarantine can save lives and doctor's fees—and easily prevent three migraines in three days.

(Postscript: The day after I wrote this, I blew my nose and immediately my sinus began to swell again. Within hours, I had my fourth migraine in five days. Two weeks later, I was still on antibiotics. Yeesh.)

NOTES

1. Charles Dickens, *Bleak House* (New York: Penguin Classics).
2. Ibid.
3. Alanis Morissette, *Jagged Little Pill*, Maverick, June 13, 1995, compact disc.
4. Charles Dickens, *Bleak House* (New York: Penguin Classics).
5. Ibid.

CHAPTER 19
BOOKS AND RESOURCES

BOOKS

A Modern Herbal: The Medicinal, Culinary, Cosmetic and Economic Properties, Cultivation and Folk-Lore of Herbs, Grasses, Fungi, Shrubs & Trees with Their Modern Scientific Uses. Mrs. M. Grieve. Volumes I & II. Dover Edition reprint, 1971. Harcourt, Brace & Company, 1931.

National Formulary. Author Unknown. University of Michigan Library reprint, 2013.

American Pharmaceutical Association, 1888.

The Rodale Herb Book: How to Use, Grow, and Buy Nature's Miracle Plants. Edited by William H. Hylton. Rodale Press, 1974.

The Complete Medicinal Herbal: A practical guide to the healing properties of herbs, with more than 250 remedies for common ailments. Penelope Ody. Dorling Kindersley, 1993.

Herbals: Their Origin and Evolution, 1470-1670. Agnes Arber. Cambridge Science Classics reprint, 1990. Cambridge University Press, 1912.

The New Garden Encyclopedia: Victory Garden Edition. Edited by E.L.D. Seymour. Wm. H. Wise & Co., 1944.

Henderson's Handbook of Plants and General Horticulture. Peter Henderson. Peter Henderson & Company, 1889.

School of Natural Healing. Dr. John R. Christopher. Christopher Publications, 1976.

ONLINE RESOURCES

SeedRenaissance.com—specializing in seeds for medicinal herbs, as well as vegetables.

Pfaf.org—an excellent resource for all kinds of garden plants, with diagrams and pictures of medicinal herbs and descriptions of some of their historic medicinal uses, among other information.

webmd.com/vitamins-supplements/default.aspx— This website includes a list of the potential interactions and side effects of medicinal herbs.

umm.edu/health/medical/altmed—The University of Maryland Medical Center's Complementary and Alternative Medicine Guide, which includes a list of the potential interactions and side effects of medicinal herbs.

Swsbm.com—Southwest School of Botanical Medicine is a rich source of information from the late master herbalist Michael Moore, based in Bisbee, Arizona.

Herbalgram.org—the website of HerbalGram, the Journal of the American Botanical Council.

MedlinePlus is a service of the U.S. National Library of Medicine, and provides a guide to herbs and supplements, including informtion about potential drug interactions: http://www.nlm.nih.gov/medlineplus/druginfo/herb_All.html

A Nievve Herball or Historie of Plantes—This is an online scanned version of the original book published in London in 1578 by Rembert Dodoens. It is fascinating.

Biodiversitylibrary.org—"A consortium of natural history and botanical libraries that cooperate to digitize the legacy literature of biodiversity held in their collections and to make that literature available for open access."

Botanical.com—an online site based on the 1931 Modern Herbal books by Mrs. M. Grieve. This site gives recipes, an index to plants, the ancient history of specific herbs, and more.

CHAPTER 20
DEFINITIONS

ANTISPASMODIC: Herbal remedy for keeping calm.

BOLUS: Herbal vaginal suppository (a method of administering medicine; *bolus* is Latin for ball or lump).

COMPRESS: A small fomentation (applied to smaller area) for relieving symptoms.

DECOCTION: Roots boiled in water for 20 minutes to extract medicinal properties.

DIAPHORETIC: Herbs used to induce sweating.

ENURESIS: uncontrolled night time urination.

FOMENTATION: Gauze or cotton soaked in an herb tea and placed on the body to heal. This is an application of the tea or herbal juice placed on the body to alleviate pain or enhance healing as well.

GLYCERITE: A glycerin tincture.

HERBAL BATH: A very hot bath infused with herbs. Use cloth tea bags for ease of clean up. Three or four bags of tea make a good herbal bath.

HERBAL STEAM TREATMENT: An herbal steam treatment is an herb, like horseradish, heated in water and placed so that the ill person can place their face above the heat and cover their head with a towel. Deep breathing is encouraged. The steam from the herb and the water will help clear mucus and sinuses.

LOZENGE: A honey-based pill (like a cough lozenge) for sucking on for medicinal benefit.

MENSTRUUM: Various liquids used to preserve quality of herbs.

OIL PREPARATION: An oil preparation is an infusion of herbs in oil.

POULTICE: Crushed herbs (sometimes in a gauze packet) placed on the body to alleviate pain or enhance healing.

SALVE: A creamy mixture made with herbs, often using beeswax, for external application.

TEA: A beverage made by covering the herbs with boiling water and steeping for 20 minutes.

BIBLIOGRAPHY

Brody, Jane. "Babies Know: A Little Dirt Is Good for You." *New York Times.* Jaunary 26, 2009. Accessed October 21, 2014. http://www.nytimes.com/2009/01/27/health/27brod.html?_r=0.

Carollo, Kim. "Pay Dirt: Hundreds of Doctors Earned Big Money from Drug Companies." October 25, 2010. http://abcnews.go.com//Health/Wellness/drug-companies-payments-doctors-revealed-database/story?id=11929217.

Christopher, John R. *School of Natural Healing.* Springville, UT: Christopher Publications, 2010.

Combest, Wendell, and George Nemecz. "Echinacea." *U.S. Pharmacist.* Accessed October 21, 2014. http://web.campbell.edu/faculty/nemecz/George_home/references/Echinacea.html.

Dickens, Charles. *Bleak House.* New York: Penguin Classics.

Diehl, J. H. "Combined Effects of Irradiation, Storage, and Cooking on the Vitamin E and B1 Levels of Foods." *Food Irradiation* 10 (April 14, 1967): 2–7.

Dioscorides, Pedanius. *Book Five: Of Vines and Wines.* Translated by Tess Anne Osbaldeston. http://www.ibidispress.scriptmania.com/index.html.

Food and Drug Administration. "FDA recommends health care professionals discontinue prescribing and dispensing prescription combination drug products with more than 325 mg of acetaminophen to protect consumers." Last updated January 15, 2014. Accessed October 21, 2014. http://www.fda.gov/Drugs/DrugSafety/ucm381644.htm.

———. "FDA limits acetaminophen in prescription combination products; requires liver toxicity warnings." Last updated January 13, 2011. Accessed October 21, 2014. http://www.fda.gov/NewsEvents/Newsroom/PressAnnouncements/ucm239894.htm.

Goodwin, Doris Kearns. *No Ordinary Time.* New York: Simon & Schuster, 1994.

Gurney, James. *Dinotopia: A Land Apart from Time.* Nashville, TN: Turner Publishing, 1994.

Herper, Matthew. "The Truly Staggering Cost of Inventing New Drugs." February 10, 2012. http://www.forbes.com/sites/matthewherper/2012/02/10/the-truly-staggering-cost-of-inventing-new-drugs/.

Hunter, Beatrice Trum. *The Natural Foods Cookbook*. New York: Touchstone, 1969.

Kendall, P. "Botulism." May 2012. Accessed October 21, 2014. http://www.ext.colostate.edu/pubs/food-nut/09305.html.

Lee, W. M., "Acetaminophen and the U.S. Acute Liver Failure Study Group: Lowering the Risks of Hepatic Failure." *Hepatology* 40, no. 1 (2004): 6–9.

"Liberty." *Webster's Dictionary 1828—Online Edition*. Accessed October 21, 2014. http://webstersdictionary1828.com/.

Linus Pauling Institute. "Garlic and Organosulfur Compounds." http://lpi.oregonstate.edu/infocenter/phytochemicals/garlic/.

McNeil Consumer Healthcare Division. "Our Story." Accessed October 21, 2014. http://www.tylenol.com/news/about-us.

Medline Plus. "Herbs and Supplements." Accessed October 21, 2014. http://www.nlm.nih.gov/medlineplus/druginfo/herb_All.html.

Morissette, Alanis. *Jagged Little Pill*. Maverick. June 13, 1995. Compact disc.

National Center for Complementary and Alternative Medicine. "Herbs at a Glance." http://nccam.nih.gov/health/herbsataglance.htm.

Natural Medicines Comprehensive Database. Accessed October 21, 2014. http://naturaldatabase.therapeuticresearch.com/home.aspx?cs=&s=ND.

NIH News. "Obesity Threatens to Cut U.S. Life Expectancy, New Analysis Suggests." March 16, 2005. http://www.nih.gov/news/pr/mar2005/nia-16.htm.

Ranasinghe1, Priyanga, Shehani Pigera1, G. A. Sirimal Premakumara, Priyadarshani Galappaththy1, Godwin R Constantine, and Prasad Katulanda. "Medicinal Properties of 'True' Cinnamon (*Cinnamomum zeylanicum*): a Systematic Review." October 22, 2013. doi: 10.1186/1472-6882-13-275.

Robbins, Carolyn. "Does a Cut-up Onion Clear Sinus?" December 18, 2013. Accessed October 21, 2014. http://www.livestrong.com/article/535180-does-a-cut-up-onion-clear-sinuses/.

Ruebush, Mary. *Why Dirt is Good: 5 Ways to Make Germs Your Friends.* Fort Lauderdale, FL: Kaplan, 2009.

Shaik, Y. B., M. L. Castellani, A. Perrella, F. Conti, V. Salini, S. Tete, B. Madhappan, J. Vecchiet, M. A. De Lutiis, A. Caraffa, and G. Cerulli. "Role of Quercetin (a Natural Herbal Compound) in Allergy and Inflammation." *Journal of Biological Regulators and Homeostatic Agents* 20, no. 3–4 (2006): 47–52. http://www.ncbi.nlm.nih.gov/pubmed/18187018%20.

St Clair, Debra. *The Herbal Medicine Cabinet.* Berkeley: Celestial Arts, 1997. University of Maryland Medical Center. "Willow Bark." Accessed October 21, 2014. http://umm.edu/health/medical/altmed/herb/willow-bark#ixzz2yX1f9Zo0.

———. "Quercetin." Accessed October 21, 2014. http://umm.edu/health/medical/altmed/supplement/quercetin#ixzz2xli9IMc2.

WebMD. "Vitamins and Supplements Center." Accessed October 21, 2014. http://www.webmd.com/vitamins-supplements/default.aspx.

———. "Willow Bark." Accessed October 21, 2014. http://www.webmd.com/vitamins-supplements/ingredientmono-955-WILLOW%20BARK.aspx?activeIngredientId=955&activeIngredientName=WILLOW%20BARK.

Zimmerman, Neetzan. "Maine Doctor Slashes Prices by Rejecting Health Insurance." May 29, 2013. http://gawker.com/maine-doctor-slashes-prices-by-rejecting-health-insuran-510289623.

INDEX

M

Ma Huang 19, 30, 37
Menstruum 51, 105
Mormon Tea 19, 30, 37
Mullein 17, 18, 19, 22, 30, 31, 36, 37, 47, 64, 84, 85–86, 92, 99, 100

N

Nervine 89, 90

O

Onion 63, 67–69, 92, 108
Oregano 3, 4, 18, 19, 31, 37

P

Peppermint 3, 15, 17, 19, 31, 32, 37, 40, 58, 74, 94, 95, 99, 101
Plantain 2, 18, 19, 21, 23, 32, 37, 78, 81, 82, 83
Poultice 36, 67, 82, 92, 105

S

Salve 1, 24, 27, 54, 77, 78–79, 83, 89, 90, 105
Self-Heal 19, 33, 38
Sinus Rinsing 8, 87–88, 99
Soapwort 20, 33, 38

Spearmint 20, 33, 38, 40
Stevia 4, 20, 34, 38, 74, 98
Stimulant 25, 28, 31, 33, 41, 58, 91, 92
St. John's Wort 15, 20, 32, 37, 42

T

Tincture 30, 37, 39, 40, 45–51, 54, 55, 57, 58, 61, 64, 74, 75, 77, 81, 82, 83, 85, 86, 88, 89, 90, 92, 93, 94, 95, 96, 99, 105
Tuning Fork 79–80

V

Valerian 15, 20, 34, 38, 40, 89, 90
Vinegar 39, 46, 47, 49, 51, 53, 54, 55, 57, 63, 64, 71–72, 96, 97

W

White Horehound 28–29, 37
Wildcrafting 20
Willow Bark 84–85, 86, 108

Y

Yarrow 20, 21, 22, 34–35, 38, 49, 64, 92, 93, 99

ABOUT THE AUTHORS

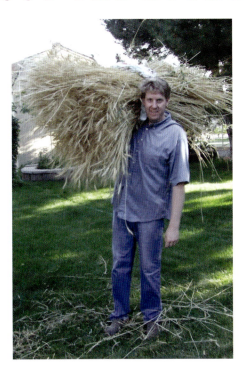

Caleb Warnock is the popular author of three nonfiction books and a novel with recipes. He has a master's degree in writing from Utah State University and a bachelor's from Brigham Young University, and he has won more than twenty awards for writing and journalism. Caleb lives with his family on the Wasatch Bench of the Rocky Mountains. He has six stepdaughters and six grandchildren. (There's no "step" between him and his grandchildren.) In his spare time, Caleb relaxes in a hammock strung between an apple and a maple tree, overlooking the perennial flowers and vegetable gardens (yes, he has more than one vegetable garden). His blog, *Backyard Renaissance*, can be found at CalebWarnock.blogspot.com. He sells pure, never-GMO, never-hybrid vegetable seeds (including some of the rarest seeds in the world) at SeedRenaissance.com. You can reach him by email at CalebWarnock@yahoo.com.

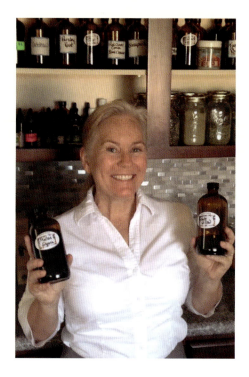

Kirsten Skirvin is a renaissance woman and master herbalist whose experience spans over twenty years. She fell in love with herbs and all their possibilities while studying edible plants for survival. She loves period costumes, large hats, aprons with pockets, and the smell of fresh flowers. The old arts call to her, demanding to be mastered, though she has yet to make a broom. She lives near the Wasatch Mountains with her amazingly supportive husband and their seven great kids.

the FORGOTTEN SKILLS of SELF-SUFFICIENCY

used by the
MORMON PIONEERS

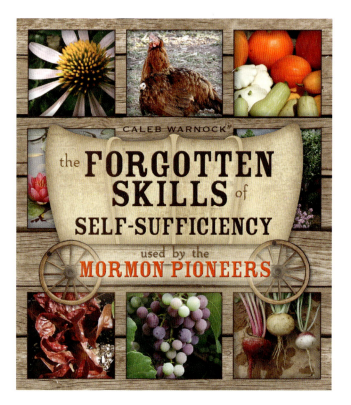

Many people dream of becoming self-reliant during these times of fluctuating prices and uncertain job security. Using truly simple techniques, you can cultivate the pioneers' independence to provide safety against lost wages, harsh weather, economic recession, and commercial food contamination and shortages. Now you can discover the lost survival skills they knew, used, and passed down for generations—skills such as how to

GROW HARDY, PERENNIAL, AND LONG-KEEPING VEGETABLES

REVIVE THE PIONEER SEED BANK

BAKE WITH PIONEER YEAST

CREATE A STRAW CELLAR

COOK WITH FORGOTTEN RECIPES

AND MORE!

THE ULTIMATE PRACTICAL GUIDE for the pioneer in all of us, this book will strengthen your family's self-reliance. Discover anew the joy of homegrown food, thrift, and self-sufficient living. Order your copy today!

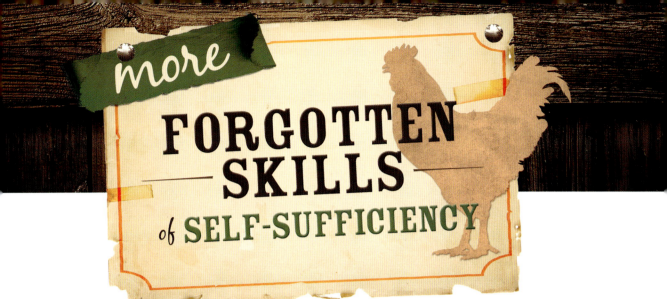

more FORGOTTEN SKILLS of SELF-SUFFICIENCY

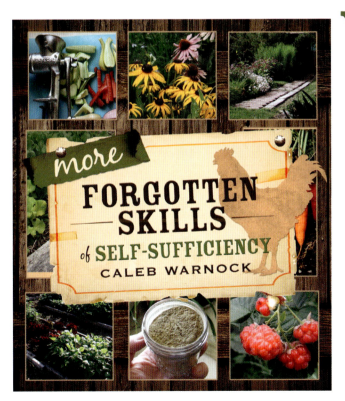

Your ancestors knew how to live self-sufficiently—now you can follow in their footsteps!

Bestselling author Caleb Warnock is back with a new collection of money-saving and healthy-living skills to help your family gain independence and self-reliance. Learn how to

GROW SELF-SEEDING VEGETABLES

BUILD RAISED GARDEN BEDS USING STEP-BY-STEP INSTRUCTIONS

COLLECT WATER FROM RAIN AND SNOW

MAKE YOUR OWN LAUNDRY DETERGENT

FIND WILD VEGETABLES FOR EVERYDAY EATING

Discover these tricks and more from the author of The Forgotten Skills of Self-Sufficiency and Backyard Winter Gardening. You can be a living example of independence for the rising generation, and avoid grocery store prices while you're at it.

Whether you're growing an organic family garden or running a no-nonsense household, More Forgotten Skills of Self-Sufficiency is a must-have guide to becoming truly self-reliant for you and your family.

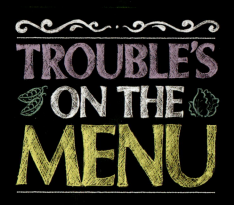

TROUBLE'S ON THE MENU

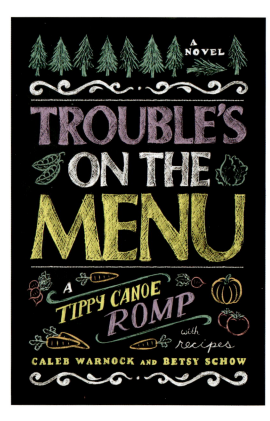

HALLIE DOESN'T BELONG in Tippy Canoe, Montana. She's a California girl used to sunshine and warmth—not cold and snow. But after the unexpected death of her estranged husband, she braves the winter weather to wrap up some of his estate details, only to discover that she doesn't fit in and none of the townspeople like her.

THAT IS, except for the town's handsome mayor, who takes quite an interest in Hallie.

BUT WHEN HIS LIFE starts to spiral out of control, she must decide if he's worth sticking around for in the long term. Join Hallie in this fast-paced, hilarious romance as she learns that sometimes love is the only remedy for a broken heart.

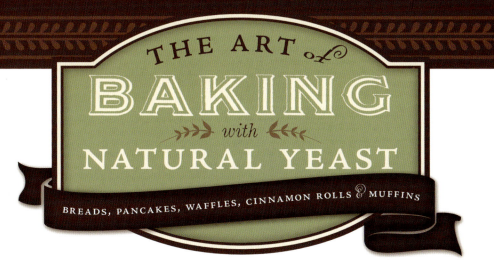

THE ART of BAKING with NATURAL YEAST

BREADS, PANCAKES, WAFFLES, CINNAMON ROLLS & MUFFINS

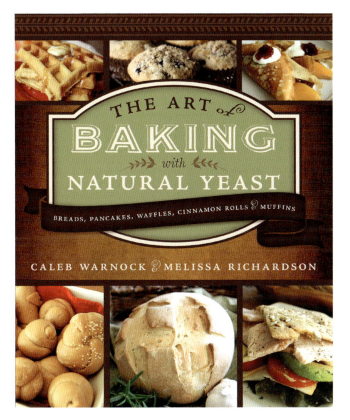

CALEB WARNOCK & MELISSA RICHARDSON

This is the book you've been waiting for! With groundbreaking information about the health benefits of natural yeast, this book will revolutionize the way you bake! Easy to prepare and use, natural yeast breaks down harmful enzymes in grains, makes vitamins and minerals more easily available for digestion, and converts dough into a nutritious food source that won't spike your body's defenses. Improve your digestive health and happiness with these delicious recipes you can't find anywhere else!

BE SURE TO TRY THE:

BLUEBERRY CREAM MUFFINS

QUICK AND EASY CREPES

GARLIC ROSEMARY SOURDOUGH

WHIMSY ROLLS

NO KNEAD BREAD

From quick and easy treats for a busy day to elaborate creations for special events, you'll find something tasty and nutritious to tempt everyone's taste buds!

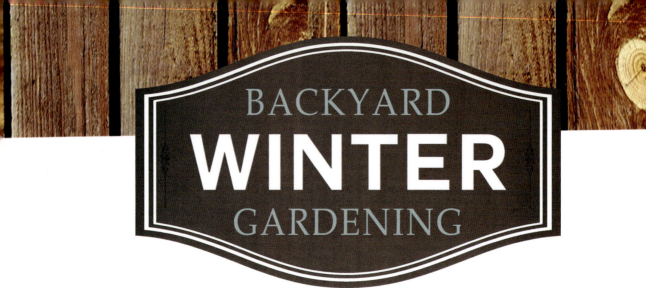

BACKYARD WINTER GARDENING

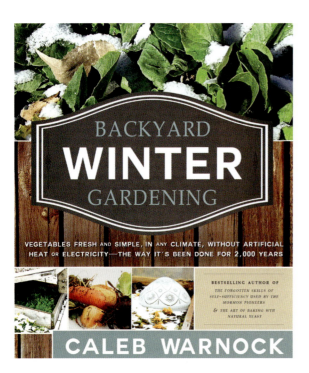

MISCONCEPTIONS ABOUT WINTER GARDENING are everywhere: that it's too difficult, slow, or even impossible. But long before the convenience of grocery stores, people in the 17th, 18th, and 19th centuries used fresh all-natural winter gardening to keep fruits and vegetables on the table even during the coldest months of the year. Feeding your family fresh food from your own backyard garden all winter long is far easier and less time-consuming than you might imagine. And you won't find better-tasting food at any price!

IN BACKYARD WINTER GARDENING YOU'LL LEARN

- how to grow winter produce without electricity, artificial heating, or lighting

- how cold temperatures don't have to result in a dead garden

- how to build a cold frame, a hotbed, and even a geothermal greenhouse for protection from harsh weather

- how children will love vegetables if they take part in the gardening

- how winter gardening protects against economic turmoil, teaches self-providence, and protects your food from unknown chemicals and contamination